The Dementia Care Workbook

Gary Morris and Jack Morris

Open University Press

Open University Press
McGraw-Hill Education
McGraw-Hill House
Shoppenhangers Road
Maidenhead
Berkshire
England
SL6 2QL

email: enquiries@openup.co.uk
world wide web: www.openup.co.uk

and Two Penn Plaza, New York, NY 10121—2289, USA

First published 2010

A catalogue record of this book is available from the British Library

ISBN-10: 0-33-523431-3 (pb) 0-33-523430-5 (hb)
ISBN-13: 978-0-33-523431-8 (pb) 978-0-33-523430-1 (hb)

Library of Congress Cataloging-in-Publication Data
CIP data applied for

Typeset by Kerrypress Ltd, Luton, Bedfordshire
Printed and bound in the UK by Bell and Bain Ltd., Glasgow

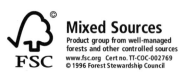

Mixed Sources
Product group from well-managed
forests and other controlled sources
www.fsc.org Cert no. TT-COC-002769
© 1996 Forest Stewardship Council

The *McGraw-Hill* Companies

To Pamela, Ben and Ruth, thank you for your support and encouragement – Jack

To Emily, Lottie, William, Sam, Daisy and Caitlin,

and

Barry Richard Morris
... gone to Nutwood

      with much love – Gary

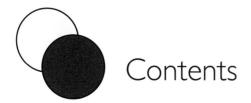

Contents

Acknowledgements

We would like here to acknowledge some of the important assistance we have received from a number of individuals and which has helped in the writing of this workbook.

Firstly, Rachel Crookes, who has been immensely encouraging and supportive as well as providing us with some very valuable feedback throughout this process – from proposal construction through to the completion of the workbook. Secondly, Jack Fray for his help and advice at frequent intervals with this project and in particular with the cover design. Thirdly, to the many healthcare students who have helped us through their engagement with our varied experiential teaching approaches in formulating structures and ideas about learning in dementia care.

Also, the authors and publishers would like to acknowledge and thank the Alzheimer's Society for their cooperation and generosity in allowing us to reproduce extracts from their *Living With Dementia* magazine, the Alzheimer's Forum and their online fact sheets. We would also like to thank the following individuals for their permission to reprint their quotes: Terry Pratchett; Yvonne Hague; Meri Yaadain; and the team at Merevale House.

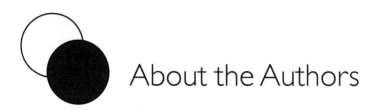 About the Authors

Gary Morris is a mental health lecturer at the University of Leeds. His practice background is in psychotherapy (cognitive analytic therapy, therapeutic community practice, psychodrama) and dementia care. He teaches on the mental health programme managing modules in dementia care and mental health issues and the media.

Jack Morris is a retired mental health lecturer from the University of Leeds. He has been involved both with educational and clinical services for individuals requiring dementia care, as well as services for people with enduring mental health problems and aspects of forensic care provision.

Introduction

This workbook builds upon the current ethos within dementia care which promotes a more person-centred approach as advocated by researchers and practitioners. The intentions are to reflect upon the reality of working within dementia care and the degree to which person-centred approaches and their accompanying theoretical and philosophical principles can be incorporated within your own practice. Acknowledgement is given to the reality of the person with dementia's living environment and the obstacles and constraints that might be encountered. Although much of this may be outside your control it is the emphasis upon reflection, problem-solving and a 'best fit' approach that we feel provides a valuable learning opportunity. It is not therefore the intention of this workbook to present you with a list of 'idealized' principles which could be difficult to achieve but more to help you reflect upon and develop person-centred approaches which are adaptable and achievable given the unique nature of your clinical practice.

A strong emphasis within this workbook is upon the quality of the relationship that is established and maintained between healthcare workers and those experiencing dementia. Consequently, we have included a range of exercises and activities which challenge some of the related interpersonal dynamics, in particular notions of *engagement* and *connectedness*. This incorporates reflection upon three distinct components: those of *self* (you the reader); the *person with dementia*; and the *environment of care*. As illustrated in Figure 1.1 we can regard the caring relationship as having a continuous flow of information between ourselves as carers (*self*) and the person with dementia, with each subsequent communication being interpreted and responded to. This is a complex dynamic where the quality of the relationship is significantly affected by what each party's perception is of the interaction taking place. For the healthcare professional this might relate to issues such as the sense of gratification received and the degree of engagement established with those we are caring for. This will serve to either motivate or discourage our subsequent responses. For the person with dementia it might simply relate to how much they feel cared for or understood by those providing care. These interactional dynamics are also strongly influenced by the nature of the environment as, for example, a calm and comfortable setting which contains personal cues will enhance the process whilst surroundings which are over-stimulating or lacking in personal items will have the reverse effect. The caring relationship is therefore seen as a complex entity helped or hindered by the particular dynamics arising from the three core elements of *self*, *person with dementia* and *environment*.

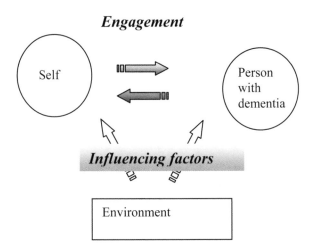

Figure 1.1 The caring relationship

Significant attention is given to examining your own practice and exploring ways in which care approaches can be enhanced, which also includes looking at issues from an organizational point of view and reflecting upon potential changes that could be made such as upgrading resources, staff training or implementing clinical supervision. Practice examples are provided through the inclusion of vignettes featuring 'Arthur' and 'Elsie', both of whom are introduced later on in this chapter. This workbook is set up so that you have the freedom to either work through material chronologically or dip into selected chapters at your leisure. Each of the chapters follows a similar structure, thereby helping you to orientate more easily with the range of concepts and dynamics under investigation and discussion. Chapters contain a number of questions, activities and exercises which allow you to contemplate and engage with specific themes. The exercises outline experiential learning approaches that we have used within classroom teaching and are presented in such a way that you can use them as part of your own learning or within a healthcare staff training programme. Full details of these are provided in Chapter 9, which considers the required resources, structure and process, as well as variations for exploring exercises from differing perspectives.

We noted in our work with healthcare students a number of problems being encountered which make it hard to match the ideals of person-centred care with actual practice. In particular, time restrictions, lack of resources, the person with dementia's level of cognitive impairment, low staff morale and the social environment itself present some of the reasons why person-centred care cannot easily be applied to practice. These problems are further maintained by the low levels of optimism already held by some healthcare students at the start of their dementia care placement, seeing it as their 'least desired option'. This caused us to look at:

- ways by which negative attitudes towards dementia care are developed or fostered;

- the degree to which theoretical principles or person-centred approaches could be realistically tied in with the realities of practice;
- ways of engaging with the *felt* and *lived* experience of those affected with dementia.

The reflective and challenging approaches adopted within our teaching sessions have been adapted and are mirrored throughout this workbook. It is expected that many of the aspects covered here have relevance to your practice experiences. This in essence addresses Alexander's (1983) 'theory–practice gap' or the 'reality shock' encountered by clinicians when trying to integrate theoretical learning with everyday practice. This workbook addresses this process by advocating a 'best fit' approach, essentially looking at how the person-centred philopsphy can be realistically adapted and applied to care. To this end we have included a number of 'best fit' tools within the following chapters linked with specific themes being discussed. These boxed items provide you with a number of suggested interventions which can be adapted and used within your practice.

Background issues

The person-centred approach to care emerged out of work carried out by humanists such as Abraham Maslow and Carl Rogers and has been used within healthcare for a number of decades. However, it is only in the last 20 years that it has begun to be applied to dementia care, advocated by individuals and groups such as Naomi Feil and Tom Kitwood/Bradford Dementia Group. The need for this type of care has gathered support and is currently promoted through a range of governmental, professional and service-user agencies. Related publications include *Living Well with Dementia: A National Dementia Strategy* (DoH 2009), the *National Service Framework for Older People* (DoH 2001), *A New Ambition for old Age* (DoH 2006a), *Dignity in Care* (DoH 2006b), *Everybody's Business* (DoH 2005) and *A Sure Start to Later Life* (Social Exclusion Unit 2005). These publications and governmental initiatives promote person-centred and individualized approaches to care. They also highlight the importance of communication and the need to adapt care interventions to accommodate the problems caused by dementia.

What is dementia?

The term 'dementia' is used to describe the symptoms that occur when the brain is affected by specific diseases and conditions, including Alzheimer's disease, or the results of a cerebral vascular accident. Dementia is progressive with symptoms gradually getting worse, something which each person experiences in their own unique way.
Symptoms of dementia include:

- loss of memory;
- mood changes;

- communication problems.

In the later stages of dementia, the person affected will have problems carrying out everyday tasks, and will become increasingly dependent on other people.

There are a number of different types of dementia which include:

- Alzheimer's disease;
- vascular disease;
- dementia with Lewy bodies;
- fronto-temporal dementia (including Pick's disease);
- progressive supranuclear palsy;
- Korsakoff's syndrome;
- Binswanger's disease;
- HIV and AIDS;
- Creutzfeldt-Jakob disease (CJD);
- multiple sclerosis (MS);
- motor neurone disease;
- Parkinson's disease;
- Huntington's disease.

There are about 700,000 people in the UK currently with dementia and this is estimated to rise to 1 million by 2025. Although mainly affecting older people there are approximately 15,000 people in the UK under the age of 65 who have dementia. There is some evidence for a genetic link, with some individuals having a higher risk of developing dementia. At present some two-thirds of people with dementia are women (Alzheimer's Society 2007).

Arthur and Elsie

We would like to introduce you to the 'constructed' individuals 'Arthur' and 'Elsie', who are different in many ways and have had their own individual lifestyle experiences, yet now share a diagnosis of dementia. They will be revisited throughout this workbook in order to better apply some of the theoretical material being considered.

Arthur

Arthur is a 55-year-old man, married with three children (ages ranging between 21 and 28). He has suffered several strokes over the past three years and a year ago was diagnosed with vascular dementia. He attends a day hospital twice weekly and has occasionally spent time in a residential facility for respite care.

Pre-diagnosis

Arthur worked as a local manager for a small transport haulage firm, having overall responsibility for 90 employees. He did not have any particular hobbies or outside interests as a large amount of his time was taken up with work, although he did attend a number of work-related social functions and conferences. He was a social/heavy drinker, consuming far in excess of the recommended weekly units, although described this as 'pressure of the job'. He was prone to stress and had been treated over the past five years by his GP for high blood pressure.

Post-diagnosis

Arthur has become increasingly dependent upon his wife Marjorie since being forced to retire from work. His short-term memory is very poor although he still retains a good awareness of past events. As a consequence he finds day-to-day experiences very confusing and quickly becomes impatient. He is prone to aggressive outbursts and bouts of weeping. Talking to Arthur is difficult as he finds it hard to maintain concentration and becomes easily distracted. This is a frustrating experience both for Arthur and those talking to him and tends to result in Arthur isolating himself from others for increased periods of time. Arthur's confusion has led him on a couple of occasions to make sexual advances towards other women whom he has mistaken for his wife. His daughter lives locally and sees him regularly, although both his sons live abroad and have little contact with him.

Elsie

Elsie is an 83-year-old woman living in a residential care home. She is a widower, her husband Sidney having died ten years ago. She has two children (Trevor and Jean) and eight grandchildren, although contact with them has steadily decreased as her condition has deteriorated. Concerns were raised when Elsie was found wandering a fair distance from her house in the early hours of the morning. She was unable to find her way home and was dressed only in her nightdress and slippers.

Pre-diagnosis

Elsie had years previously worked as a veterinarian, her passion for animals evident in the range of pets (dogs, cats and budgerigars) that she and Sidney had kept at their house. After her retirement, Elsie had been very keen on outdoor pursuits and had with her husband been a member of a rambling club. She enjoyed meeting other people and had a very active social life. When not engaged in these activities she would content herself with word puzzles and crosswords as a way of 'keeping my mind sharp'.

Post-diagnosis

Elsie has fluctuating periods of lucidity and confusion, becoming extremely distressed when she is more aware of her deteriorating cognition (on one occasion she was found by healthcare staff screaming and shouting obscenities). She rarely gets involved with activities and poor concentration and confused thinking have made crosswords and word puzzles very difficult. Her mobility is poor and she has fallen on a number of occasions. She is also periodically incontinent (sometimes doubly), her poor orientation and levels of confusion causing problems. She rarely leaves the residential home and seldom now has visits from her family, partly as they are often a distressing and confusing experience for all concerned.

Workbook chapters

Following this Introduction the book is divided into eight further chapters, as follows.

The felt experience: the *person* with dementia

The experience of dementia as seen by those encountering this condition first hand.

The felt experience: carers

The carer's perspective as related to partners and other family members.

Attitudes

The notion of *double discrimination* – age and dementia related.

The environment of care

The significance of a person's environment (own home or practice setting) upon their overall sense of well-being.

The *person* with dementia

The unique individual within person-centred care.

Engagement: connecting with the *person*

Forming a connection with those experiencing dementia.

Empowerment and disempowerment

Autonomy and risk-taking within dementia.

Facilitating person-centred care: worksheets and activities

Facilitating group working and experiential exercises.

Conclusion

While recognizing some of the very real obstacles presented in practice, this workbook essentially aims to encourage the best care possible. Engagement difficulties can be experienced through the communication or cognitive deficits of the person with dementia, our own limitations in delivering care, as well as the restrictions posed by the environment itself. It is our intention that through sampling and working through the theoretical content and activities provided in each chapter you will be able to consider the 'best fit' for your own practice area, thereby maximizing the extent to which person-centred care can truly be applied.

References

Alexander, M. (1983) *Learning to Nurse: Integrating Theory and Practice.* Edinburgh: Churchill Livingstone.

Alzheimer's Society (2007) *Dementia UK: The Full Report.* London: Alzheimer's Society.

DoH (Department of Health) (2001) *National Service Framework for Older People.* London: DoH.

DoH (Department of Health) (2005) *Everybody's Business. Integrated Mental Health Services for Older Adults: a Service Development Guide,* http://olderpeoplesmentalhealth.csip.org.uk/ everybodys-business.html, accessed 8 July 2008.

DoH (Department of Health) (2006a) *A New Ambition for Old Age,* www.dh.gov.uk/en/ Publicationsandstatistics/Publications/PublicationsPolicyAndGuidance/DH_4133941, accessed 10 September 2008.

DoH (Department of Health) (2006b) *Dignity in Care,* www.dh.gov.uk/en/Policyandguidance/ Healthandsocialcaretopics/Socialcare/Dignityincare/index.htm, accessed 10 September 2008.

DoH (Department of Health) (2009) *Living Well with Dementia: A National Dementia Strategy.* London: DoH.

Social Exclusion Unit (2005) *A Sure Start to Later Life,* www.cpa.org.uk/cpa/ seu_final_report.pdf, accessed 25 October 2008.

Further reading

Feil, N. (1993) *The Validation Breakthrough: Simple Techniques for Communicating with People with 'Alzheimer's-Type Dementia'.* Baltimore, MD: Health Professions Press.

Kitwood, T. (1997) *Dementia Reconsidered: The Person Comes First.* Buckingham: Open University Press.

Maslow, A. (1970) *Motivation and Personality.* London: Harper & Row.

Rogers, C. (1961) *On Becoming a Person: a Therapist's View of Psychotherapy.* Boston, MA: Houghton Mifflin.

2 The felt experience: the *person* with dementia

Objectives: After reading this chapter you should be able to:

➡ Reflect upon what the experience of dementia feels like for those directly affected.
➡ Discuss the impact that a diagnosis of dementia has upon those concerned.
➡ Reflect upon the concerns and fears facing those with dementia.

Clinical problems (the person with dementia's perspective)

'I'm struggling, I know something's wrong but I feel too embarrassed and frightened to tell anyone.'

'I know I get agitated but nobody really listens. I just receive more medication.'

'I'm not always given clear information or properly involved within my own care.'

'When I'm no longer able to express myself and make my needs known, will anyone care?'

'And yet … if I am assisted to express myself and feel understood by those offering care I will be better able to cope.'

Introduction

This chapter, along with Chapter 3, addresses the experience of dementia from a *felt* and *lived experience*, drawing directly upon the perspectives of those concerned. This chapter examines the experience of those who are affected directly by dementia, and Chapter 3 deals with the experience of carers (family members and friends). The term *felt experience* can be understood as the emotions and thoughts encountered and refers essentially to a person's inner world and the way in which progressive changes are personally experienced. It can be regarded as a unique journey which differs from person to person according to a variety of individual factors. Looking at these helps to address the question, 'What does it feel like?' with regards to actually living with dementia and all its associated aspects.

Understanding what a person affected with dementia might be experiencing depends upon the extent to which:

- they are able to express themselves;
- we are able or willing to listen.

The ability to express oneself can be hindered by numerous factors of which cognitive decline is only one. Accompanying physical or mental health problems play a significant part – for example, aphasia (as a result of strokes) or withdrawn and subdued behaviour borne out by the presence of depression. We must also consider the fact that the generally low expectations directed towards those who are aged or have dementia may result in individuals having poor self-confidence and finding it hard to communicate their wishes for fear of rejection or dismissal by others. As a person's expressive ability deteriorates others tend to make more assumptions about what they are thinking, what they are feeling and what their needs might be.

Activity 2.1

It might be assumed that people in the later stages of dementia don't have feelings or logical thoughts.

➡ What do you think of this statement?

When considering the extent of feelings or logical thought held by those in the later stages of dementia it is imperative to recognize that they are still sentient and unique human beings. A person's inability to verbally communicate emotions such as fear or anger does not mean that these feelings are absent. Indeed, if we look more carefully at a person's facial expressions, gestures, tone of voice and overall behaviour, many clues will become apparent as to their underlying emotions and thoughts. More attentive listening allows a person's behaviour to be more correctly understood within its total context and our subsequent responses become more person-centred. For example, while aggressive or agitated behaviour might be commonly treated through pharmaceutical or behavioural interventions, it might be more beneficial to look at the antecedents such as underlying feelings of threat, helplessness and frustration.

The awareness of what another person is *actually* experiencing in terms of how they understand their world is something that we attempt to ascertain, although the degree to which we are able to do this can be questioned. Specific terms are used within healthcare work to denote the process of connecting with another's inner experience. These include the interpersonal approaches of *empathy* and *validation* which encourage an appreciation of another's unique perspective. Understanding what a person with dementia might be experiencing or feeling allows us to respond more appropriately and sensitively. It requires us to find out what is happening at each stage in a person's journey from the initial shock of diagnosis through subsequent changes caused by a progressive deterioration in cognitive functioning. Of course, each person is unique and our understanding of the dementia experience gathered through previous engagements with others is not necessarily transferable. Another aspect to bear in mind is the extent to which our understanding might be based upon assumptions or a sense of how *we* might feel if placed in another person's position. This projects our personal frame of reference directly into the mind of another person with no guarantee of securing a match. It is the way in which a lifetime's experiences, memories and feelings fit together as a *whole* that is important, along with the unique way in which these impact upon a person. This means that each event in a person's life has meaning that transcends a single experience. We might for example find it hard to understand why a frail elderly woman is rejecting our help until we find out that she has always been a strongly independent woman and is striving to maintain a sense of control and purpose.

Not understanding another person's felt experience means that there is the potential for interventions to be ineffective. For example, we might identify that a person is isolated and withdrawn and encourage their involvement in group activities. However, the reasons why social contact is avoided can be multi-faceted and for some people with dementia may relate to feeling overwhelmed and exhausted by trying to attend to extensive amounts of stimuli (Davis 1989; Bryden 2005). What we would need then are activities that help to accommodate this problem, offering contact but in a more manageable and acceptable way. Therefore, in order to best support the person with dementia we need to look at ways to facilitate their expression as well as maximizing our ability to hear what they have to say.

Where do we get our information from?

Activity 2.2

➡ Write down the different types of source we can access in order to find out what a person's felt experience of dementia entails.

When considering the *felt experience* it is important to understand what this means as what we learn from available research studies or person-centred literature has the tendency to keep us at a distance from what a person actually experiences within their day-to-day existence. From these sources we learn of aspects such as increased isolation, despair, depression and anxiety as a consequence of a deteriorating level of cognition. It is when we meet and talk with people with dementia or access first-person accounts that we truly begin to understand the significance and resonance of what dementia sufferers are living through. This is where we are invited in to share something of the person's experience in its full context and the feelings evoked such as extreme frustration and humiliation felt at the recognition of personal deficits and losses, or the sometimes cruel and harsh treatment by others. Terms such as 'despair' are better understood when related to events such as Larry Rose's (1996) painful and humiliating struggle with cognitive assessment tests and his realization that he was unable to complete simple activities which he reflected his 5-year-old grandchild could easily accomplish. This highlights the point that the most important source of understanding about the dementia experience is from those most directly affected – individuals who are in a unique position to help us understand better what they are encountering. Meeting with people encountering dementia and speaking face to face with them about what they are living through is perhaps the prime approach to take, although this can be complemented by studying documented first-person media accounts. Surprisingly, despite the richness of this personal resource for learning about dementia, it has remained relatively untapped by researchers (Downs 1997; Woods 1997). This reflects something of the discriminatory approach and sense of low expectations that are generally directed towards those with dementia, with their personal accounts not being afforded due validity and credibility.

Our understanding of the lived experience of dementia therefore comes from personal or family experience, direct contact through a professional caring role and the accessing of various media products (see Figure 2.1) such as literature and poetry, television documentaries, film depictions and postings on internet sites. Utilizing first-person material concerning mental health problems presents a valuable source of learning for healthcare professionals (Oyebode 2003). This view is supported by Vassilas (2003), who stresses the importance for clinicians of accessing literary accounts of dementia in order to understand more of the condition and its real impact upon people's lives. There are critics though, such as Wolpert (2003), who states that it is potentially too difficult to accurately describe one's feelings of mental health problems and that these accounts probably help other sufferers more than they do those treating them. This is a fairly dismissive viewpoint and fits in with the generally low expectations already afforded the mentally ill, particularly so in the case of those with dementia. What we need to recognize is that each individual, no matter how cognitively impaired, has an expressive ability and the fault in comprehension may lie more with our inability to facilitate communication or to 'hear' what is being related. The more we attempt to tune into the person with dementia's world or access their personal accounts the more perceptive and questioning we will become about the needs of those we are caring for. Most of the available first-person accounts relate to earlier experiences of dementia, when individuals retain more of an expressive ability. With the later stages of dementia it becomes difficult to get much more than a glimpse of what the experience really feels like for those directly affected. There is a need therefore to increase our understanding and develop techniques and approaches that facilitate and recognize further expression.

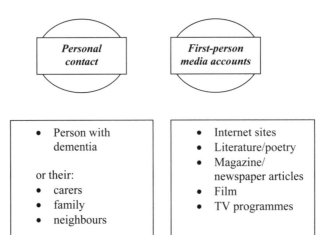

Figure 2.1 Learning about the dementia experience

Activity 2.3

Have a look at the following first-person accounts of living with dementia.

➡ Bryden (2005) *Dancing with Dementia*
➡ Davis (1989) *My Journey into Alzheimer's Disease*
➡ Friel-McGowin (1993) *Living in the Labyrinth*
➡ Rose (1996) *Show Me the Way to Go Home*

Tuning in

Exercise 1: Watching Iris

This exercise provides an insight into the impact that the condition of dementia has upon a couple – the person with dementia and their partner/carer. It also addresses the ways in which their relationship together is affected. We have provided you with details about conducting this exercise in Chapter 9.

Healthcare students were asked to watch *Iris*, a film which illustrates the progressive cognitive deterioration as experienced by the writer Iris Murdoch. It reflects upon her life before and after the disease as well as the strain upon the relationship with her husband John as they both struggle to cope. The students were given questions to consider at three distinct stages: before, during and after watching the film. It is worth noting here that prior preparation for this exercise involved a number of introductory sessions around the topic of dementia. Students appeared notably moved by this film and commented on how they felt powerfully engaged with Iris and her husband John, understanding more about the experience involved and picking up a strong sense of emotions such as frustration, anger and isolation. As well as the impact upon both individuals, observations were made about how they were affected as a couple and their subsequent relationship together. The potency of this exercise was apparent within student evaluations which highlighted it as one of the best features of the dementia care module.

The felt experience

The exploration of the person's felt and lived experience of dementia will be addressed with regards to the following themes:

- receiving a diagnosis ('something's wrong');
- setting out on a journey;
- struggling;
- coping ('I'm still here').

Receiving a diagnosis ('something's wrong')

The first inkling a person has that there might be something wrong can be very disconcerting and frightening, and in a number of instances they might cope by assigning difficulties to causes such as stress from work, family pressures or simply the onset of old age. Early indicators include forgetfulness, disorientation, language and motor problems, confusion, depression, agitation, inattention and getting lost (La Rue et al. 1993). The approach taken by many individuals in the early stages is to engage in strategies that deny their failings in an attempt to maintain a veneer of normality (Keady and Nolan 1995). Larry Rose (1996) in his book *Show Me the Way to Go Home* describes the perplexity and strangeness of getting lost on the drive to his mountain cabin, a route he had taken many times before, and ending up a few hundred miles away. Instead of getting to the cabin he spent the night in a motel feeling exhausted, stupid, afraid and with a 'cold frightening emptiness'. He felt reluctant to talk to others about this incident as they would think he was 'losing it', although he felt an unnerving sense of doubt stirring inside: 'I felt the uncertainty of a person experiencing a tornado for the first time; the terrifying sensation that comes on realizing that what should be firm and solid is no longer so, and cannot be relied upon' (1996: 4). Likewise, Diana Friel-McGowin (1993) writes about the disorienting and distressing experience of getting lost after dropping off her husband's lunch and spending four hours driving around (on what should have been a 20-minute trip), struggling to recollect the name of the town she lived in. She also describes problems in balancing, experiencing the floor heaving and swaying and having to cling to the wall for support.

A fascinating example is provided by Bernlef's (1988) first-person style fictional account *Out of Mind*, which chronicles the experience of Maarten, an elderly Dutchman with dementia. As his ability to construct sense and meaning from his external world starts to recede, there is a mirroring in the style of prose which becomes progressively more fragmented and distorted. It is written in the spirit of Swift's (1889) *Tale of a Tub* – in the 'language of madness' or more precisely the language of dementia. We get an impression very early in the book that something is wrong through Maarten's sense of perplexity, which gives way gradually to a more deep-seated unease. His thoughts relate that his memory has never been good although there is a blossoming sense of denial: 'Year by year things happen to your body ... this is different. More a general feeling of unease than a specific symptom. But no it would be nonsense to think there is something really wrong' (Bernlef 1988: 20).

The general reluctance to accept or acknowledge what might be going on can also be colluded by friends, family or even healthcare professionals. This is evident when it comes to presenting a diagnosis, as there may be a feeling that individuals would be better off not knowing, needing to be protected from the full impact that the results of brain scans and cognitive function assessments bring. It is hard to properly conceive what it must feel like to be told that you have dementia and how this news is subsequently acted upon. We might naturally assume that for many individuals this diagnosis comes as a huge shock, leaving them very fearful and uncertain about the future. The resultant impact though is obviously dependent upon a variety of factors including a person's level of cognitive impairment and ability to comprehend what they are being told. It is apparent that in a number of instances people are only partially or not at all informed about their condition. This is borne out by studies that show that although carers are nearly always told the diagnosis the person with dementia is not because of an assumption about their inability to understand or the concerns about the detrimental impact a diagnosis might have upon them. One such concern relates to the destroying of hope and the raised potential for suicide or depression (Pinner 2000). There are also worries about the threat that the giving of a diagnosis might have upon a person's flagging competence and fragile defences (Woods *et al.* 2003). As a consequence, diagnostic information is presented to a number of individuals through general euphemisms such as 'memory difficulties' (Downs *et al.* 2002; Bamford *et al.* 2004). The holding back of information, whilst done paternalistically, can be criticized because of the person's fundamental 'right to know' as well as not allowing them the opportunity to engage in future planning such as a 'once in a lifetime holiday' (Pinner 2000). A number of actual responses to the diagnostic process are included in Box 2.1. These reveal very mixed experiences with some receiving information through clear and supportive explanations and others encountering insensitive and negative approaches. What stands out though is a wish and need to be included within this process.

Box 2.1 Alzheimer's Forum: how I was given my diagnosis

'When we went to see the consultant, they talked to my wife while I was doing the tests. I find it insensitive and insulting. I'm not stupid – I can understand what they are saying.'

'They were lovely to me when I was doing the tests, then they called me in and explained everything to me. I think I knew what they were going to say anyway because I had been through it with my mother.'

'Why is it that when we realise we have a problem with our memory and go to the doctor, some of them are reluctant or even disinclined to include us in the consultation diagnosis of dementia. They seem to think it's better we don't know and start talking over our heads to our partner and family.'

'Please talk openly, straightforward and truthfully to me as well, then I can try to get my life into some sort of control and readjustment.'

'Grant me the respect and dignity to be able to understand and deal with my diagnosis.'

(Alzheimer's Society 2008a)

What is significant about the responses in Box 2.1 is the level of expressiveness and understanding that many people have at the point of diagnosis. Whilst desire or ability to know more about one's condition will clearly differ from person to person we should not make assumptions. It is also worth bearing in mind that reluctance to talk about a diagnosis can be due to being in denial, something that Bryden (2005) regards as being a perfectly normal response to the shock of diagnosis. Along with struggling to come to terms with a diagnosis is the difficulty of having to 'come out' to family and friends. Diana Friel-McGowin (1993) writes about the strong desire to unload her burden to others and receive support and understanding, yet being held back through feelings of embarrassment. The need to address the topic of dementia more openly and reduce the degree of stigma attached is stressed in the *Out of the Shadows* report (Alzheimer's Society 2008b). Terry Pratchett, who has himself been diagnosed with dementia and is very much involved with it states that:

> The first step is to talk openly about dementia because it's a fact, well enshrined in folklore, that if we are to kill the demon then first we have to say its name … Names have power like the word Alzheimer's; it terrorizes us. It has power over us. When we are prepared to discuss it aloud we might have power over it. There should be no shame in having it yet people still feel ashamed and people don't talk about it.

(Pratchett 2008: 8)

This statement underlines the need to confront the topic of dementia by replacing the collaborative silence with a more open and accepting exchange of views. It means helping not only individuals but couples as well to create a joint construction which enables them to make sense of their situation, manage losses and adjust to the changes experienced in roles and identity (Robinson *et al.* 2005). Recommendations for giving a diagnosis are provided in Best Fit 2.1.

Activity 2.4

➡ What do you think a person might be feeling when given a diagnosis of dementia?
➡ When do you feel people shouldn't be told?
➡ How should the diagnosis be given?

> **Best Fit 2.1**
>
> When giving a dementia diagnosis:
>
> - Don't *assume* the person doesn't want to know.
> - Treat the person with sensitivity and dignity.
> - Explain details slowly and clearly.
> - Check understanding.
> - Provide written information or links to support networks as necessary.

The steady changes taking place can cause acute frustration and distress with regards to ways in which individuals perceive themselves or feel that they might be treated or regarded by others. Of significance is what particular deficits or problems mean or represent to each person. Hamdy and Hudgins (1998) give the example of individuals in the early stages of Alzheimer's attempting to conceal their incontinence by hiding soiled clothes or wearing towels in their underwear. This is evidently a response to feelings of shame and embarrassment and the uncertainty about others' responses. Problems such as this can overshadow the *whole* person and help engage stereotypical constructs of the elderly and those with dementia, with more attention placed upon deficits and inabilities than what the individual is actually still able to do.

 Activity 2.5

Write down what you might be feeling if:

➡ You have (for the first time) been incontinent of urine.
➡ You are no longer able to drive.
➡ You struggle to find the words for everyday objects.
➡ You cannot concentrate sufficiently to watch television or read.

Activity 2.5 asked you to consider how you might feel if having to accommodate certain deficits or problems within your life. You might have included feelings such as fear, anger, frustration, embarrassment, grief or sadness. Although not necessarily providing an exact fit with others' experiences we can certainly start to appreciate something of the emotions involved. One of the main problems perhaps is the predominant focus upon *deficits*, as the term dementia commonly causes a person to be overshadowed by their condition. As Sabat (2001) states, this has a direct impact upon self-esteem as those with dementia are more often noticed for what they can't do rather than what they can do. We can suppose here that the person experiencing dementia directly becomes what we might denote a *dementia sufferer*, devoid of successes, pleasant experiences and new learning. It is important to anticipate and become aware of difficulties but it is perhaps equally imperative that we recognize and encourage attempts and opportunities to enhance a person's sense of well-being. As strongly stated on the Alzheimer's Forum: 'Being diagnosed with dementia does not mean the end of life. We still have brains, we can still laugh and cry. We still have feelings!' (Alzheimer's Society 2008a).

Setting out on a journey

The process post-diagnosis is initially one of profound shock, although later becoming a period of contemplation, where individuals try to make sense of what is happening to them and attempt to plan for the future. For some, there is the sensation of embarking on a journey, which involves venturing into the unknown. The Alzheimer's Society publishes a monthly online magazine entitled *Living with Dementia* which contains factual advice and personal experiences. One edition contained the following account, 'Navigating the sea of dementia':

> *Like Columbus, I am on a voyage of discovery. My route is not exact and I must make adjustments as I go along … unlike being at sea in a storm, I know that the voyage is only going to become more difficult. It may become a typhoon or hurricane, depending on where it takes me. This storm will not pass: I have to make suitable preparations before the force 12 hits. Let me tell you that I am lucky: I have very good friends who will be with me on the stormy ride ahead.*
>
> (Voyager 2005: 2)

Activity 2.6

➡ What do you think of Voyager's statement?

What we pick up from Voyager's statement is an awareness that things are set to deteriorate and a need to plan for certain eventualities. The desperateness of Voyager's situation is eased somewhat through the reassurance of having the support of 'good friends', no doubt individuals who can help to provide a sense of connection and grounding when things get worse. The need for continued support and personal advocates is echoed by Friel-McGowin (1993: 53): 'What I needed was someone to assure me that no matter what my future held, they would stand beside me, fight my battles with me, or if need be, for me.' The significance of these sentiments is reflected by Harman and Clare's (2006) study which investigated illness representations in early-stage dementia and found two overarching themes of:

- It will get worse
- I want to be me

The sense of impending decline is something that causes much concern as individuals contemplate comparisons with their earlier self or with peers who are functioning better. It means having to consider the impact of changes forced upon them such as having to retire from work or stop driving. The deterioration in functioning and enforcement of change is joined by the fear of losing a sense of self. This is where the support of 'good friends' or family is so vital: to have other people around who still retain a sense of *what it means to be me* when this has faded or disappeared from one's own awareness. An aspect that stands out starkly from the range of personal accounts available such as Voyager's is the level of cognitive functioning a person has the moment such feelings are expressed. As a person's condition becomes more advanced and the elements for them stormier and more tempestuous, we may only catch the odd glimpse of the vessel in the distance until it is finally engulfed in a last huge wave and lost to sight. It is the later stages of dementia that seem less accessible to us when a person becomes increasingly more isolated in their own strange and unfathomable world, unable to reach out or be accessed by others. When trying to map out a person's journey, individuals and carers might be assisted by certain 'rough' guides as to the stages of dementia (see Box 2.2). These basically regard individuals as moving steadily through a series of levels, each with a further marked level of decline until their eventual death.

Box 2.2 Stages of Alzheimer's disease

Stage 1: no impairment
Stage 2: very mild decline
Stage 3: mild decline
Stage 4: moderate decline (mild or early-stage)
Stage 5: moderately severe decline (moderate or mid-stage)
Stage 6: severe decline (moderately severe or mid-stage)
Stage 7: very severe decline (severe or late-stage)

(Alzheimer's Association 2006)

The stages illustrated in Box 2.2 can be condensed further to illustrate the following:

- mild – 'setting out on a journey';
- moderate mixture;
- severe – unable to communicate.

The 'stage theory' approach is criticized by Kitwood (1997) among others as being somewhat reductionist by not reflecting the person's individual response to dementia. Some people, he argues, move backwards and forwards between these stages as well as presenting aspects of self that represent more than one stage. The stage theory approach also does not help in determining what individuals *can do* as the focus tends towards deficits and what they *cannot do*. Indeed, Christine Bryden (2005) found herself in a downwards spiral, struggling with many activities, giving up driving, no longer answering the phone or watching television, hallucinating and becoming more depressed. She regarded herself at this point as reaching the moderate level of deterioration. She then noticed things changing as her mood state improved and she felt less confused, which led on to her resuming driving and then signing up for a degree course in theology.

Some researchers have attempted to look at stages from a different perspective, highlighting the impact on the person concerned. An example of this is Keady and Nolan's (1995) nine-stage model of dementia.

- *Slipping* (minor lapses in memory and behaviour).
- *Suspecting* (incidences become more frequent and individuals suspect something could be amiss).
- *Covering up* (conscious and deliberate attempts made to compensate for difficulties or to hide from others).
- *Revealing* (difficulties shared with those closest).
- *Confirming* (acknowledgement of the problem is made and confirmed with the diagnosis).
- *Surviving* (later changed to *maximizing*) (strategies engaged in to maximize time which the person has left).
- *Disorganization* (cognitive difficulties and associated behavioural problems become an increasingly dominant feature).
- *Decline* (caring demands are increased and residential care may be required).
- *Death* (the final stage for the sufferer).

Struggling

This section will be explored by looking at the impact caused to the person in terms of loss. This is where the person begins to struggle as a consequence of what they have already lost, are in the process of losing or are contemplating losing in the future. The struggle to come to terms with these losses affects each person in different ways, for some having very serious and profound implications including an increased risk of suicide. Key point 10 of the *Older People and Suicide* report (Beeston 2006: 27) states:

> It may be the case that Dementia is a risk factor for suicide in older people early in the course of the disease, when insight and the ability to plan and act are still present. Later in the course of the Dementia the presence of the disease may be protective insofar as insight may be lost, the ability to plan suicide and act on the plan may be severely diminished, and there may be increased levels of supervision from carers and relatives.

Therefore, it should not be assumed that individuals will necessarily begin to cope or come to terms with their condition and every effort should be made to allow individuals to express themselves and negotiate what types of support might be helpful.

Activity 2.7

➡ Faced with a future of declining cognitive ability, what do you feel are the most significant losses experienced?

As indicated, central to the many aspects affecting the person with dementia is a profound sense of loss. We can look at this in relation to Harman and Clare's (2006) themes: 'it will get worse' and 'I want to be me', where the issue of loss is profoundly featured in what a person is subsequently unable to do as well as perhaps the most frightening aspect, that of losing a sense of self. A summary of some of the core losses and the impact upon the person is illustrated in Figure 2.2.

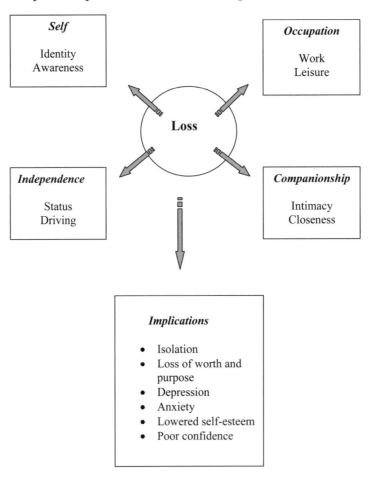

Figure 2.2 Loss

We can take some sub-themes from those featured in Figure 2.2 which encompass the core aspects being addressed. These are a loss of:

- self;
- occupation;
- independence;
- companionship.

Self

There are a number of characteristics that define who we are, borne out of the richness of many years of experience. Losing a sense of self can be contemplated as having our identity slowly stripped away. An aspect that causes much debate and something that is notoriously hard to ascertain relates to the point in a person's deterioration when for example 'I cease to be me'. Kitwood's (1997) notion of personhood and Naomi Feil's (1993) principles of validation assert the uniqueness and worth of each person irrespective of the level of deficit currently being experienced. They stress that even in the later stages when a person is (seemingly) wholly unresponsive and dependent on others for all of their care needs, the essential person within still remains. One can only imagine the torment of knowing that precious memories such as births, weddings and achievements are slipping away. There is a real sense of tragedy in knowing that a time may come when our whole family or lifetime achievements become lost to us as our cognitive abilities recede. It is in the earlier stages that individuals are prone to depression and despair as periods of lucidity make it hard to contemplate the enormity of what is happening. As reasoning diminishes the pain of loss subsides for the person, yet remains with family members and friends. The poignancy of this is starkly expressed by John Bayley concerning his wife Iris Murdoch's progressive loss of awareness: 'She does not know that she has written twenty-seven remarkable novels, as well as her books on philosophy; received honorary doctorates from all the major universities; become a Dame of the British Empire ... ' (Bayley 1999: 41).

Where we haven't had contact with individuals at a point before the condition of dementia manifested itself, the experience of individuals in the public arena perhaps enables us to comprehend something of the impact upon them from what has changed or been lost. This is very evident when considering those who have reached a high level of prominence in their chosen field, yet in later years struggled with increasing infirmity and cognitive decline (see Figure 2.3). This glittering array of talent includes people who in their prime commanded a high degree of attention and respect from others. We find them later struggling to maintain a sense of dignity or purpose, unaware of past glories or momentous events in history. This is not to belittle the experience of the non-celebrity, who in the eyes of partners, children, grandchildren or friends can be every bit as esteemed and valued for the qualities and attributes they too possessed. Recommendations for helping to maintain a sense of self are provided in Best Fit 2.2.

Best Fit 2.2

Help the person maintain a sense of self:

- By compiling a life history/review.
- By collating photographs of significant people and experiences.
- By gathering significant objects and resources.
- By running reminiscence activities.
- By maintaining optimum contact with family and friends.

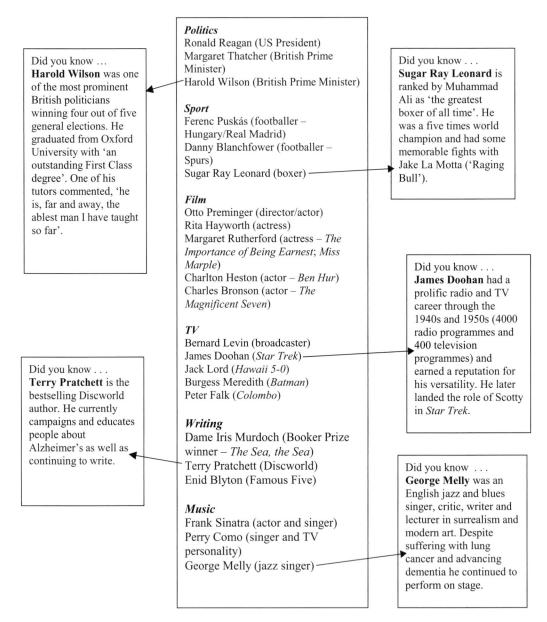

Did you know …
Harold Wilson was one of the most prominent British politicians winning four out of five general elections. He graduated from Oxford University with 'an outstanding First Class degree'. One of his tutors commented, 'he is, far and away, the ablest man I have taught so far'.

Politics
Ronald Reagan (US President)
Margaret Thatcher (British Prime Minister)
Harold Wilson (British Prime Minister)

Sport
Ferenc Puskás (footballer – Hungary/Real Madrid)
Danny Blanchfower (footballer – Spurs)
Sugar Ray Leonard (boxer)

Film
Otto Preminger (director/actor)
Rita Hayworth (actress)
Margaret Rutherford (actress – *The Importance of Being Earnest; Miss Marple*)
Charlton Heston (actor – *Ben Hur*)
Charles Bronson (actor – *The Magnificent Seven*)

TV
Bernard Levin (broadcaster)
James Doohan (*Star Trek*)
Jack Lord (*Hawaii 5-0*)
Burgess Meredith (*Batman*)
Peter Falk (*Colombo*)

Writing
Dame Iris Murdoch (Booker Prize winner – *The Sea, the Sea*)
Terry Pratchett (Discworld)
Enid Blyton (Famous Five)

Music
Frank Sinatra (actor and singer)
Perry Como (singer and TV personality)
George Melly (jazz singer)

Did you know . . .
Sugar Ray Leonard is ranked by Muhammad Ali as 'the greatest boxer of all time'. He was a five times world champion and had some memorable fights with Jake La Motta ('Raging Bull').

Did you know . . .
James Doohan had a prolific radio and TV career through the 1940s and 1950s (4000 radio programmes and 400 television programmes) and earned a reputation for his versatility. He later landed the role of Scotty in *Star Trek*.

Did you know . . .
Terry Pratchett is the bestselling Discworld author. He currently campaigns and educates people about Alzheimer's as well as continuing to write.

Did you know . . .
George Melly was an English jazz and blues singer, critic, writer and lecturer in surrealism and modern art. Despite suffering with lung cancer and advancing dementia he continued to perform on stage.

Figure 2.3 Celebrities with dementia

Occupation

Our occupation and chosen leisure pursuits are significant in helping to define who we are. They also provide us with important avenues for socialization, status and building self-esteem. Having to give up these activities because of increased difficulty or stress will have a major effect upon the person concerned. The ability to continue with previously engaged occupations is dependent upon a variety of factors including a person's level of functioning, the degree of support available and the particular demands of the activity. Although diagnosed with dementia, the author Terry Pratchett has stated his intention to continue writing, asserting that there was 'time for a few more books yet' (BBC 2007). The Jazz singer George Melly continued to perform despite suffering with advancing dementia. However, many others are forced into early retirement as the demands of their chosen profession become unmanageable. Robert Davis (1989) for example relates the pain and anguish at having to relinquish his role as pastor of a large church. Likewise, Diana Friel-McGowin (1993) writes about the torturous process of giving up work in her mid-forties because of increasingly making mistakes. She coped at first by taking temp work in different offices where mistakes or confusion could be more easily explained away but finally had to take early retirement. This proved a massive blow to her self-esteem and confidence. Perhaps occupations which require greater degrees of organized and coherent thought are more difficult to maintain whereas those in creative professions, with sufficient support, are able to work for longer. Occupational recommendations are provided in Best Fit 2.3.

Best Fit 2.3

- Encourage involvement with previous hobbies and leisure interests.
- Offer opportunities for purposeful engagement.
- Make realistic adjustments to environment to maximize occupational involvement.

Independence

The steady and cumulative impact caused by loss of function or role means that individuals become more dependent upon others. It is something that can be acutely marked by those affected: 'I live with the imminent dread that one mistake in my daily life will mean another freedom will be taken from me. Each freedom taken places me in a smaller playpen with a tighter ritual to maintain myself' (Davis 1989: 103). What comes across clearly here is the decrease of personal control and an emerging sensation of powerlessness and helplessness. A particularly significant and symbolic loss of independence is caused by having to give up driving. One respondent on the Alzheimer's Forum (Alzheimer's Society 2008a) noted:

> *Recently I have been told that I can no longer drive my car as I crashed in into a keep left sign. I have fought heaven and hell to reinstate it but to no avail. Alas the decision is final and I have no choice. I just feel so angry and humiliated that I can no longer drive myself around, instead I rely on my children and personal friends.*

It is a statement which highlights some common themes concerning the contemplation of diminishing independence with a resultant drop in worth, self-esteem and freedom.

Case Study 2.1 Arthur

To recap: Arthur is a 55-year-old man with vascular dementia who previously worked as a local manager for a small transport haulage firm with overall responsibility for 90 employees. He has poor short-term memory which causes him to become easily impatient and distressed.

Arthur

It is absolutely galling to feel so utterly stupid and helpless as well as to have to put up with the intolerance and insensitivity of others. I went to buy a paper from the local newsagent's yesterday which I do every day in order to keep a bit of independence. I don't walk too well and tend to stumble a bit and need to hold onto things to help keep my balance. I overheard someone say, 'It's a bit early to be drinking isn't it?' which made me very angry and upset. I was so affected by this that I lost my bearings and couldn't find my way home. After wandering around for about an hour I did finally stop someone to ask for directions but couldn't remember my address. He was very unsympathetic and walked away, leaving me feeling stupid. I was fortunate though that my wife Marjorie had been out looking for me and picked me up in our car. This has shaken me up so much I just want to stay at home now and shut the world out.'

Case Study 2.1 looks at what loss of independence means to Arthur. His experience is symbolic of many people with dementia and shows how even those who were previously confident and capable can start to feel a sense of unease with the world and wish to retreat away. This is reflected by Bob Davis (1989), a person with Alzheimer's who recounts being panic stricken and distressed in large crowds despite previously being very confident in public. Part of his struggle related to coping with the proliferation of stimuli which quickly made him confused, having to sit down and regroup his thoughts. Shopping centres with uneven lighting and crowds moving in different directions disoriented him and the sight of row after row of produce in supermarkets left him feeling exhausted. Exposure to experiences such as these were completely draining, necessitating time alone (often days) to recover. Therefore, in order to help maintain independence we need to recognize what a person's limits are and achieve a balance between over-stimulation and under-stimulation. It means carefully listening to the person and pitching activities at a level they can productively cope with. Further recommendations are provided in Best Fit 2.4.

Best Fit 2.4

- Identify opportunities for independent activity.
- Look into available resources and aids that assist independent living (i.e. Telecare).
- Create a safe environment where mistakes or slow performance can be supported.

Companionship

Restrictions in social experience coupled with a progressive loss of companionship can promote a profound sense of loss. This is in part caused by the uncertainty and discomfort felt by the person with dementia as well as others who feel unsure as to what to say and how to respond. As observed by Larry Rose (1996: 32): 'I am becoming more and more withdrawn. It is so much easier to stay in the safety of my home ... than to expose myself to people who don't understand, people who raise their eyebrows when I have trouble making the right change at the cash register, or when I'm unable to think of the right words when asked a question'. The outcome of experiences such as these is that people lose much of their former social confidence and become very isolated. These issues form a specific focus for support agencies and have led to the setting up of a range of projects to keep people connected. In Leeds, West Yorkshire, for example services include contact and information points from the Alzheimer's Society, the Community Links Home Support Service, Volition (supporting voluntary service groups) and Together: Working for Well-Being (advocacy, assertive outreach and intensive support). There are also web-based agencies aimed at keeping people connected – for example, the Alzheimer's Forum whose internet site enables people with dementia to have contact with others in similar circumstances, thereby helping to combat feelings of isolation and the sense of being alone with one's problems. This is a worthy and important venture, especially given the advantages of this medium with its 24-hour access and anonymity of use (Brown 2002), however deficits in internet access and computer familiarity can limit its use. Companionship recommendations are provided in Best Fit 2.5.

Best Fit 2.5

- Provide opportunities for people to talk about their companionship needs.
- Discuss options for social contact.
- Look for available resources and activities (i.e. web forums, dementia cafes).

Exercise 2: Understanding behaviour

Students were given a chapter of Robert Davis's book *My Journey into Alzheimer's Disease* to read and asked to answer the following questions:

- What sense do you make of the difficulties experienced by the narrator?
- How might these affect his subsequent behaviour or response towards others?
- Consider ways in which he could be best supported to cope with these difficulties.

The selected chapter, 'The abnormal changes so far' focused specifically upon the difficulties he was experiencing such as paranoia, fear of making mistakes, poor concentration, agitation, wandering behaviour, disorganization, sleep problems, quickly feeling overwhelmed and a need for rituals and routines. Accessing his inner thoughts and feelings enabled students to be more aware about the types of underlying issues that impacted upon his subsequent behaviour – for instance, using rituals to manage anxiety or withdrawing from social contact when feeling overwhelmed. Discussion then related to clinical practice and the different types of experience that might be behind so called *challenging behaviours* like agitation or sexual disinhibition. The importance of this activity was the encouragement for students to consider possible causes or influences for all behaviours that are observed. This enabled them to develop interventions that supported the person within their experience as opposed to simply managing the behaviour displayed. Full details of this exercise are provided in Chapter 9.

Coping ('I'm still here')

To contrast against the difficulties noted in the previous section it is important to understand some of the ways that people with dementia learn to cope with their condition. Part of this comes from a sense of acceptance, a point at which energy can be focused upon maximizing remaining resources and abilities. Peter Ashley received a diagnosis of dementia with Lewy bodies and initially struggled to accept it, but after opening up about his feelings felt encouraged to fight on, make the most of his life and return to some form of work (Alzheimer's Society 2008c). The determination to make the most of life despite having a diagnosis of dementia is stressed by Larry Rose: 'There is so much to do, so little time ... I am going to live every minute like it was my last' (1996: 127). This sentiment is reflected by many others as evidenced within posted information on the Alzheimer's Scotland (2003) website (see Box 2.3). These feelings challenge the stereotypical view of the person with dementia as helpless and incapable.

Box 2.3 I am a person with dementia

'Being diagnosed with Alzheimer's disease is not the end of the world, whilst appreciating that things have changed, there's still a whole world to enjoy.'

Pat

'Dementia is not a major part of your life, just part of it. I don't wake up with my first thought being "I have dementia!" I plan ahead and wake up thinking of the activities I have arranged to do that day.'

James

'Same person? – no, I'm a better person, I now have a greater understanding of impairments.'

Ian

(Alzheimer's Scotland 2003)

Harman and Clare (2006) reflect the coping stance taken by those experiencing dementia as lying on a continuum between self-maintaining responses (aimed at maintaining the prior sense of self and seeing problems as a normal part of ageing) and self-adjusting responses (acknowledging the changes dementia brings and integrating them into one's sense of identity). This helps to shift the focus from a *deficits-led* perspective to what might be regarded as an *abilities-led* approach. It strongly communicates a personal message of 'I'm still here' as a reminder that the attachment of a diagnostic label has not robbed the person of the fact that they still have much to offer or achieve. An excellent illustration of this can be seen with Christine Bryden's (2005) heartening example of her struggle to be received as a credible advocate of people with dementia. She shows us by example that it is possible to have a profitable and satisfying life post-diagnosis, meeting and marrying her husband, speaking regularly at conferences and actively campaigning for better understanding about the experience of dementia. Her brave, coherent and eloquent prose can be seen in sharp contrast to what one might imagine perhaps from somebody diagnosed with dementia. This is not to say that as the condition advances she won't struggle to get her thoughts heard. What is evident is the desire by people with dementia to be taken seriously and be listened to, to be received credibly and to be treated with dignity and respect. Examples such as these provide hope for others with dementia. Whilst not ignoring the fact that life is often hard or that they also have moments of despair and extreme frustration, they importantly help to balance this with reflections about the abilities they do have and the reserves that in some cases they did not know they had. The emphasis here is upon maximizing potential and of living one's life to the full, in some instances making the person more productive and fulfilled post-diagnosis.

The increased number of individuals with dementia, earlier detection rates and active campaigning mean that the public have an enhanced visibility of those who are still at an optimum stage of functioning. Another salient factor is the increased utilization of person-centred approaches and better social and psychological care practices which foster *rementing* processes (Sixsmith *et al.* 1993; Kitwood 1997). We might also look at new improved treatment regimes including the use of drugs such as Aricept (donepezil) which helps to maintain function and well-being among those with Alzheimer's-type dementia and mild to moderate degrees of impairment (Birks and Harvey 2006).

It is especially hard for those who are able to express themselves with a degree of lucidity and as a result are discredited as not really having *proper* dementia or being unrepresentative of others with this condition. As more people are diagnosed at earlier stages (or due to the fact that there are more opportunities for self-expression) the way many people present themselves does not match the generally held dementia stereotype which views individuals in later stages unable to communicate or care for themselves. An example of a person being 'written off' or discredited because of their dementia is provided in Case Study 2.2.

Case Study 2.2 Elsie

To recap: Elsie is an 83-year-old retired veterinarian with Alzheimer's disease. She previously had an active social life and a wide range of hobbies/interests. These have been hindered by her lack of contact with family and friends, poor mobility and periods of confusion.

Elsie

'I know I have periods of confusion where my head seems filled with fog and I can't think very clearly, but a lot of the time I feel fine. I write poetry and small stories, I like doing word puzzles and I still enjoy talking to people. I get told sometimes that I seem perfectly normal and don't seem to have much wrong with me – which is true. Dementia for me is a hindrance but not a compete disability. At other times though people seem to get hung up on the word dementia and expect me to be gaga. It shows how little they know, only able to picture the latter stages of this illness. Just because I'm 83 and have dementia doesn't mean I should be written off. I'm still here damn it!'

Conclusion

There are surprisingly a large number of means which provide access to the inner world of those experiencing dementia. The restrictions that limit this process are both actual and assumed, caused through dynamics as diverse as stereotypical expectations or the level of a person's impairment. As covered in Chapter 4, expectations of both the elderly and those with dementia are generally low. It is interesting to note here how the way in which we see others or how they see themselves can undergo a dramatic transformation following the allocation of a diagnosis. This is synonymous with the concept of *labelling*, where all of a person's behaviours are subsequently interpreted in the light of that label (Becker 1963). This is also true of individuals experiencing dementia where forgetfulness and poor concentration caused by stress or anxiety are taken as further evidence of their failing cognitive ability. Therefore, understanding another's inner world takes a lot of skill, time and patience in order to properly interpret and piece together their total experience.

Key points

- 'When you regard me, notice what I *can* still do, not just what I *can't*.'
- 'Please include me as much as possible within the process of care.'
- 'Involve me when presenting a diagnosis of dementia.'
- 'When I am no longer able to make my wishes known, treat me still with dignity and respect.'
- 'Please excuse my failings and be patient with me.'

References

Alzheimer's Association (2006) *Stages of Alzheimer's Disease*, www.alz.org/AboutAD/Stages.asp, accessed 29 June 2006.

Alzheimer's Scotland (2003) *'I'll Get By with a Little Help from my Friends'*, www.alzscot.org/downloads/friends.pdf, accessed 10 January 2008.

Alzheimer's Society (2008a) Alzheimer's Forum, www.alzheimersforum.org/site/index.php, accessed 17 April 2008.

Alzheimer's Society (2008b) *Dementia: Out of the Shadows*, www.alzheimers.org.uk/downloads/Out_of_the_Shadows.pdf, accessed 31 March 2009.

Alzheimer's Society (2008c) *Living With Dementia*, www.alzheimers.org.uk/site/scripts/documents.php?categoryID=200241, accessed 15 November 2008.

Bamford, C., Lamont, S., Eccles, M., Robinson, L., Mar, C. and Bond, J. (2004) Disclosing a diagnosis of dementia: a systematic review, *International Journal of Geriatric Psychiatry*, 19: 151–69.

Bayley, J. (1999) *Iris: A Memoir of Iris Murdoch*. London: Abacus.

BBC (2007) *Author Pratchett has Alzheimer's*, http://news .bbc.co.uk/1/hi/entertainment/7141458.stm, accessed 13 December 2008.

Becker, H. (1963) *Outsiders: Studies in the Sociology of Deviance*. New York: The Free Press.

Beeston, D. (2006) *Older People and Suicide*. Stoke-on-Trent: Centre for Ageing and Mental Health, Staffordshire University.

Bernlef, J. (1988) *Out of Mind*. London: Faber & Faber.

Birks, J. and Harvey, R. (2006) *Donepezil for Dementia due to Alzheimer's Disease*, www.cochrane.org/reviews/en/ab001190.html, accessed 22 May 2006.

Brown, H. (2002) Information for patients, in B. McKenzie (ed.) *Medicine and the Internet*, 3rd edn. Oxford: Oxford University Press.

Bryden, C. (2005) *Dancing with Dementia*. London: Jessica Kingsley.

Davis, R. (1989) *My Journey into Alzheimer's Disease*. Buckinghamshire: Tyndale House.

Downs, M. (1997) The emergence of the person in dementia research, *Ageing and Society*, 17: 597–607.

Downs, M., Clibbens, R., Rae, C., Cook, A. and Woods, R. (2002) What do general practitioners tell people with dementia and their families about the condition? A survey of experiences in Scotland, *Dementia: The International Journal of Social Research and Practice*, 1: 47–58.

Feil, N. (1993) *The Validation Breakthrough: Simple Techniques for Communicating with People with Alzheimer's-type*. Baltimore, MD: Health Professional Press.

Friel-McGowin, D. (1993) *Living in the Labyrinth: A Personal Journey through the Maze of Alzheimer's Disease*. New York: Delacorte Press.

Hamdy, R. and Hudgins, L. (1998) Urinary and fecal incontinence, in R Hamdy, J. Turnbull, J. Edwards and M. Lancaster (eds) *Alzheimer's Disease: A Handbook for Caregivers*, 3rd edn. St Louis, MO: Mosby.

Harman, G. and Clare, L. (2006) Illness representations and lived experience in early stage dementia, *Qualitative Health Research*, 16(4): 484–502.

Keady, J. and Nolan, M. (1995) Assessing coping responses in the early stages of dementia, *British Journal of Nursing*, 4: 309–14.

Kitwood, T. (1997) *Dementia Reconsidered*. Buckingham: Open University Press.

La Rue, A., Watson, J. and Plotkin, D. (1993) First symptoms of dementia: a study of relatives' reports, *International Journal of Geriatric Psychiatry*, 8: 239–45.

Oyebode, F. (2003) Autobiographical narrative and psychiatry, *Advances in Psychiatric Treatment*, 9: 265–71.

Pinner, G. (2000) Truth telling and the diagnosis of dementia, *British Journal of Psyciatry*, 176: 514–15.

Pratchett, T. (2008) *Living with Dementia*, www.alzheimers.org.uk/site/scripts/documents.php?categoryID=200241, accessed 15 November 2008.

Robinson, L., Clare, L. and Evans, K. (2005) Making sense of dementia and adjusting to loss: psychological reactions to a diagnosis of dementia in couples, *Aging and Mental Health*, 9(4): 337–47.

Rose, L. (1996) *Show Me the Way to Go Home*. Forest Knolls, CA: Elder Books.

Sabat, S. (2001) *The Experience of Alzheimer's Disease: Life Through a Tangled Veil*. Oxford: Blackwell.

Sixsmith, A., Stilwell, J. and Copeland, J. (1993) Dementia: challenging the limits of dementia care, *International Journal of Geriatric Psychiatry*, 8: 993–1000.

Swift, J. (1889) *The Tale of a Tub and Other Works*. London: Routledge.

Vassilas, C. (2003) Dementia and literature, *Advances in Psychiatric Treatment*, 9: 439–45.

Voyager (2005) Navigating the sea of dementia, www.alzheimers.org.uk/I_have_dementia/PDF/Newsletter/Livingwithdementia_Jan2006.pdf, accessed 12 May 2006.

Wolpert, L. (2003) Invited commentary on autobiographical narrative and psychiatry, *Advances in Psychiatric Treatment*, 9: 270–1.

Woods, B. (1997) Talking point: Kitwood's 'The Experience of Dementia', *Ageing and Mental Health*, 1: 11–12.

Woods, R., Moniz-Cook, E., Lliffe, S., Campion, P., Vernooij-Dassen, M., Zanetti, O. and Franco, M. (2003) Dementia: issues in early recognition and intervention in primary care, *Journal of the Royal Society of Medicine*, 96: 320–4.

3 The felt experience: carers

Objectives: After reading this chapter you should be able to:

➡ Discuss how the condition of dementia and its associated characteristics can have an emotional drain on the carer and significant others.
➡ Explore how the carer's duality of roles can be influenced by changes in living environments and a generalized deterioration in health.
➡ Reflect upon how a person's dementia can influence the feelings, thoughts and behaviours of carers.

Clinical problems (the carer's perspective)

'It was a relief to find a nursing home for my husband as it just became too hard for me to continue looking after him. I can't help feeling guilty though.'

'I sometimes feel so angry with my mother. I know I should control my temper more but I get so frustrated with her.'

'My partner and I made so many plans for the future ... all the things we would do together once we both retired. I just feel cheated.'

'And yet ... with proper support and opportunities to express and work through my feelings I would find it easier to cope.'

Introduction

This chapter explores the impact that the condition of dementia has upon the lives of informal carers and family members. It focuses upon the range of issues and conflicting emotions they have to contend with as they proceed through various phases from initial diagnosis through to the death of a loved one. Their caring role is at times immensely stressful and is often referred to with the phrasing 'burden of care' as individuals have to contend with feeling helpless, exhausted, guilty and lonely. Coping with excessive demands and pressures with variable levels of support can severely impact upon the physical and mental health of carers as well as resulting in abusive or aggressive behaviour being displayed towards those they are caring for. At times carers are confronted with enormous emotion-laden decisions, perhaps none more so than when relatives have to move into residential care. Although they might initially feel some relief and reassurance that others are now going to take up the caring role there are also complicated feelings of guilt and failure to contend with. Although much of the caring experience comprises difficulties and problems it is worth recognizing that positive elements can also be found. These includes feelings of closeness with those they are caring for or an enhanced sense of purpose through being needed. It is the totality of this experience with its multi-varied elements, negative and positive, that will be explored within this chapter.

In many instances carers have a duality of roles and will be both family members and carers. They are individuals who predominantly assume the role of caring for another person not because it is their job to do so but because of love and concern for that person (i.e. partners or children). While dementia *carers* might be widely expected to consist of elderly partners looking after ailing spouses, the reality is that carers could be children, nephews/nieces, grandchildren, cousins, friends or neighbours. A point to stress here is that even those who are not directly involved with the care situation (the wider family, for example) will have their own issues to contend with, notably feelings of guilt or loss. The current increase in individuals being diagnosed with dementia at younger ages (i.e. HIV/AIDS or alcohol related) does not preclude relatives from older generations such as parents having to reprise their former caring role with their children. However, within this chapter, for ease of reference, the role of carer as *partner* will form the main consideration. It is worth noting though that the experience of being a carer may have commenced some time before the emergence of any recognizable dementia symptoms because of other health needs or relationship dynamics.

Sources of information

The experience of carers has been drawn from a number of sources including research articles and various media products such as internet sites, books, television documentaries, radio programmes, films, newspaper articles and magazine features. The internet in particular offers carers a platform for sharing their own experience as well as gaining comfort from others' postings and the realization of not being alone. A notable example here is the chat-room style format provided by the Alzheimer Society's Talking Point forum.

Activity 3.1

➡ Have a look at the Alzheimer's Society's Talking Point Forum (an online community for people with dementia and their carers, family and friends to discuss all aspects of the condition).

www.alzheimers.org.uk/talkingpoint/site/index.php

There are sometimes ethical or moral objections with regards to the recounting of 'real life' experiences. For example, the biographical account *Iris* was criticized for being written while Iris Murdoch was still alive, making it potentially unjustifiably intrusive and prying. The debate according to Vassilas (2003) relates to the degree to which a person's illness should be described. However, *Iris* provided a powerful spotlight upon the carer's perspective and the very real impact that the illness of dementia has upon a partner and some of their resultant feelings such as frustration, rage, isolation and despair.

The carer's experience

Before addressing some of the main issues for carers it would be useful for you to first consider your own thoughts as to some of the difficulties they face. This is addressed in Activity 3.2.

Activity 3.2

What do you feel are the main difficulties experienced by carers regarding the following perspectives?

➡ Emotional
➡ Sociological
➡ Physical
➡ Psychological

When contemplating the experience of carers you might have thought about the physical and emotional strain they are under, the variable degrees of support available and the feelings of isolation they may experience. Certainly, the carer's role can at times be an extremely burdensome and stressful task as many cope with unmanageable degrees of pressure yet receive little or no support. Carers are prone to feeling isolated and have to contend with their own physical and mental health problems while still having to provide 24-hour care with little or no respite. In many cases, carers' needs tend to be overlooked unless they present with some type of health crisis themselves. The experience facing carers incorporates many different types of problem. This varies significantly from person to person and we should consider certain features such as the relationship between the carer and those cared for, their ages and health state, environmental factors and the type and nature of resources available. Although some might readily take on the role of carer, others do it with resentment and trepidation. This may in part be governed by the degree and types of support available. The carer's experience can be better understood through accessing some of the many first-person accounts available. Exercise 3.1 details the use of the Internet as an information resource.

Exercise 1: Internet guided study – 'the lived experience of carers'

This guided study is outlined in detail in Chapter 9 and provides insights into the actual felt and lived experience of dementia as encountered by carers. It involves visiting the internet site of the health charity group 'healthtalkonline' and completing a related worksheet. This site features carers' responses to issues including:

- getting the diagnosis;
- wandering;
- arranging residential care;
- driving;
- money;
- living with change;
- complicated emotions;
- end of life.

The interviews are accessible as transcripts, audio files or videos. Students we offered this guided study to reported subsequently being more mindful about carers with an awareness that it was easy for their needs and feelings to be overlooked. This highlighted the need for carers to have their experience addressed along with that of the person with dementia.

Core issues

A carer's experience is obviously strongly influenced by the stage and severity of a person's dementia and the degree to which their lives are affected. We can consider for example the concern and confusion felt as early symptoms become apparent as well as the sense of shock when receiving the diagnosis. The impact upon carers from physical and psychological demands can be severe. Whatever personal time a person has may be fleeting with an unwelcome return soon after to the role of carer. It is in some ways reminiscent of the exhausted mother's experience, trying to cope with the 'demands' of a highly dependent child. However, there is consolation for the mother via small signs of change – for example, the child begins to sleep for longer periods throughout the night. For the carer the reverse may be true with increasingly disturbed or unsettled behaviour being demonstrated. Each day becomes more and more unpredictable with many difficult and arduous encounters still lying ahead. It is perhaps inappropriate to try and itemize the carer's experience through distinct stages although a very rough approximation can be addressed as follows:

1   First signs/diagnosis
2   The burden of care
3   Carer abuse
4   Social isolation
5   Finding meaning and joy from caring

6   Moving into residential care
7   Facing the end

First signs/diagnosis

The first signs of dementia can be hard to detect and may be passed off as overwork, stress or a consequence of other physical ailments. It is obviously an immense shock to all concerned when a diagnosis of dementia is confirmed, bringing with it many associated fears and fantasies. As reported in the TV documentary *Malcolm and Barbara* (ITV1, 8 August 2007), when Barbara received her husband's diagnosis: 'the word [dementia] rang round and round in my head, almost like a death sentence'. This illustrates something of the devastating impact that a diagnosis of dementia has. When confronted with the initial diagnosis of dementia it is hard to imagine exactly how individuals and their families feel about and cope with their sense of shock and disbelief. A fair proportion of what is already 'known' about dementia might be based upon assumptions and erroneous facts. There is clearly at this stage a very real need for information, reassurance and support. The extent to which this is fulfilled and the manner in which individuals are informed of their diagnosis is unclear. As seen in Chapter 2 it appears to be a very variable process with carers tending to be given more details than those they are caring for, a number of whom feel poorly informed.

Activity 3.3

➡   Write down what you think the initial feelings might be for the carer, family members and friends following a diagnosis of dementia.
➡   When might it be necessary to tell other people?
➡   What information would it be relevant for the carer to give?

Coping with the shock of diagnosis is extremely difficult and requires having to consider major changes to one's life and in a number of instances necessitates a premature retirement from work. The multitude of conflicting feelings, allied with the level of stigma associated with dementia, makes it hard to know how and what to tell others – be they family, friends or associates. It is also worth considering that the rise in younger-onset dementia and earlier detection rates means that a number of working-age adults are having to contemplate living with a condition which they had previously assumed only affects the very old. A glimpse at this process is provided by Yvonne Hague's moving statement about her husband's dementia which was posted on the Alzheimer's Society's website. What is particularly poignant here is the ages of those concerned – a time of life where a diagnosis of dementia is not expected.

Box 3.1 Your story – Alzheimer's Society

My childhood sweetheart

Yvonne Hague

It is hard to think that the person most dear to me, my soulmate, was diagnosed with dementia.

Knowing that my father-in-law was diagnosed at 49 and passed away at 53 is no comfort as here I am at 39 trying to come to terms with the fact that my beloved partner of 23 years (my childhood sweetheart and father to my 10-year-old daughter) was diagnosed at 40 with moderate to severe dementia.

Emotionally it is crippling me and physically I am trying to keep my full-time job going to keep home and family together. My darling husband has chosen in his mind to block out the diagnosis presented to him in March this year and feels he is absolutely fine. But given the negative start to this letter I do not wish you to feel that I am giving up or struggling to find positives in daily life.

I try to create memories for us as family and try to keep positive but I cannot convey how little information or support there is for young people affected by dementia. I want to know how others cope and how I can influence the local services in a way that is of value to my husband.

He is and still remains the person I married, just with a very poor memory. His character and spirit is still there and he continues to tell me that he loves me every day. Rightly or wrongly my daughter has not been told the full extent of her daddy's condition because I know that she is not strong enough at present because she is still dealing with the death of her grandfather.

Juggling work, the needs of my daughter and those of my husband is my biggest hurdle. This is truly a catch 22 situation for me.

(www.alzheimers.org.uk/site/scripts/documents_info.phpdocumentID=590)

Activity 3.4

➡ How do you feel when hearing about younger people being diagnosed with dementia?

➡ What services or self-help organizations do you know of for young people?

The diagnosis of dementia is currently being made at earlier stages and in some cases before symptoms have fully manifested. While an individual retains many faculties and abilities and to most intents and purposes appears to be the same person, it can be very hard to accept the validity of their diagnosis (Butcher *et al.* 2001). There is a sense of incongruity presented where a person has health problems which are not immediately observable. Rebecca Stevenson (2007: 17), writing about her father's Alzheimer's disease, noted remarks from others at a party: ' "Your dad's doing so well, you'd never know he had anything wrong with him", although he was standing in a corner on his own because he wasn't able to make a connection with what people were talking about.' Likewise, in the television documentary *Malcolm and Barbara*, Barbara remarked about her husband: 'on the surface he looks as though he's the same person but you know inside there's something eating him away and depriving me of the person I knew and love'. A feature here for carers concerns how much to reveal to people they encounter during the normal course of each day – for example, shop assistants, restaurant workers or bus drivers, in order to 'excuse' or 'accommodate' any subsequent inappropriate or difficult to manage behaviour. Unlike the person with a more visible ailment, dementia is a condition which in the early stages can remain undetected by others not familiar with this individual and therefore unable to make sufficient allowances for how they subsequently behave. For example, a person might be holding up a supermarket queue while struggling to use a credit card for payment and in the process evoking impatient or abusive remarks from others. While informing others can be helpful it can also prove distressing and arduous for carers, especially as their reaction may not always be sensitive or helpful.

The burden of care

Activity 3.5

If you had the responsibility of caring for a relative with dementia who requires significant help with self-care needs, is periodically verbally aggressive and demanding, is unaware of who you are and at times very disoriented, how might this impact upon:

➡ Your own health?
➡ Your social network (friends)?
➡ Your future aspirations?

There are a number of studies that have been carried out highlighting the burden of care endured by carers of relatives with dementia, such as Schulze and Rössler (2005) or Kjellin and Östman (2005). These stress some of the profound difficulties and feelings encountered by those coping with what seems to be unbearable and unmanageable degrees of stress. For many carers there seems little respite, an experience which is very different to the role of professional carers where care is delivered in allotted times. The continuous process of care is so demanding that Mace (1992) refers to the perception of a 36-hour day. The position facing carers is hard, feeling torn between loyalty and love for their relative and doubts about their ability to cope. Indeed, in Archbold and Stewart's (1996) study, 80 per cent of caregivers reported that they were willing to make substantial sacrifices in order to continue caring for a family member at home for as long as possible. Some of the driving factors as to why family members are willing to take on the caring role (Eisdorfer 1991) relate to:

- love or reciprocity;
- bonds maintained over many years;
- recognition that others would provide the same care if the positions were reversed.

Alternatively, Brodaty et al. (2005) indicate that the role may be strongly influenced by guilt or as a response to social pressure. Clearly those in the latter group will suffer more stress and resent their role to a greater degree. Dementia has been described as an unremitting burden on the family (Anderson 1987) and caring for a person with a chronic mental health condition is more stressful than caring for a person with a physical disability or disorder. Prolonged dementia care leads to caregiver strain with psychological, physical, social and financial implications (Gallagher et al. 1989; Coope et al. 1995; Samuelsson et al. 2001) and Mittelman et al.'s (1995) study found significant numbers of carers meeting the diagnostic criteria for depression. The physical effects can be significant, with increased access to healthcare being sought, and are even associated with a higher mortality rate (Schulz and Beach 1999). Tabak et al.'s study (1997) revealed that the most difficult behaviours for carers to cope with were aggressive behaviour, sleeplessness and verbal and behavioural repetition

Exercise 2: A day in the life

We invited two carers to share their experience of living and coping with a partner who had dementia with a group of healthcare students. This approach follows the structure found in a number of magazines and newspapers where individuals are asked to document a typical 'day in the life'. It highlighted very starkly the pressures facing carers as well as the wider family. For ease of writing, the day was broken into three parts: morning, afternoon and evening. However, it should be noted here that for many carers the day is prolonged with many disrupted nights: to avoid being too intrusive, night-time details were not requested. Carers were provided with the opportunity to share their account with a small group of students with space for questions and discussion following each of the designated three parts. What came across from this presentation was the potency and expressiveness of the stories shared and how the students engaged with the profound sense of the very real difficulties and feelings involved. Learning opportunities such as this provide us with an appreciation of what the carer's experience is of living and coping with a partner and their dementia. This takes us beyond initial responses such as 'I'm struggling' or 'I'm not coping very well' and allows us insights into what these expressions actually signify. This is where we start to understand the fuller context and realize something of Mace's (1992) concept of the 36-hour day. What is vital is that practitioners become more mindful of the support needs of carers who are hopefully then not so easily overlooked, with more effective support subsequently being offered. Details of this exercise are provided in Chapter 9.

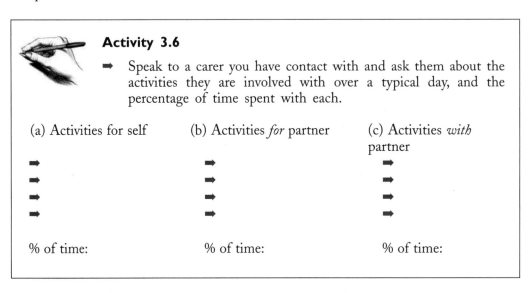

Activity 3.6

➡ Speak to a carer you have contact with and ask them about the activities they are involved with over a typical day, and the percentage of time spent with each.

(a) Activities for self   (b) Activities *for* partner   (c) Activities *with* partner

➡   ➡   ➡

➡   ➡   ➡

➡   ➡   ➡

➡   ➡   ➡

% of time: % of time: % of time:

A particular issue for many carers concerns the restricted amount of space that they have for their own needs, which generally become relegated behind those of the individuals they are caring for. There may also be feelings of guilt when attending to one's own needs with the sense that a dependent partner is being neglected. A most profoundly difficult emotional stressor facing carers concerns feelings of guilt that are evoked when they are struggling to cope or sensing that they might be letting their partner down. As you can see in Box 3.2 there are many factors which can give rise to feelings of guilt, such as getting frustrated or angry, wanting space for oneself or having to contemplate residential care. As noted by one of the respondents in Tabak *et al.*'s (1997: 88) study of carers: 'how can I get angry at him? I am an awful person and a lousy caregiver'. This reflects the conflict faced by many carers whose own needs are put to one side and have few avenues open to express and deal with their own feelings of frustration or helplessness. Recommendations for supporting carers are provided in Best Fit 3.1.

Box 3.2 Factsheet: caring for someone with dementia and dealing with guilt

Are you feeling guilty …

… because other carers seem to manage better than you do?

… because of how you treated the person before they were diagnosed?

… because you sometimes have unpleasant thoughts and feelings?

... because you sometimes get angry or frustrated?

... because you sometimes want time for yourself?

... because of feelings from the past?

... because you feel you shouldn't be accepting help?

... because you feel you can't balance all your commitments?

... because you sometimes feel trapped?

... because you've decided that the person needs to move into residential care?

... after the person's death?

(Alzheimer's Society 2008)

Best Fit 3.1

- Provide space for carers to express their feelings and concerns.
- Look at support which can be offered for psychological, social and physical needs.
- Consider appropriate and meaningful respite breaks which can be had.
- Help carers to appreciate that it is OK to not be perfect or to take time for self.

Carer abuse

Activity 3.7

➡ In what ways do you think individuals with dementia might experience abuse from their carers?

➡ What factors do you feel might precipitate carers acting abusively?

Extreme and prolonged stress coupled with exhaustion, helplessness and lack of support results unsurprisingly in a number of cases of individuals becoming angry or aggressive. There are many different types of abuse experienced by those with dementia including:

- physical;
- psychological;
- verbal;
- neglect.

It is unclear as to what the extent of abuse from carers is, although a study by Cooney and Mortimer (1995) found 55 per cent of carers reporting some type of abuse, with verbal abuse being the most common form. In contrast, Kurrie *et al.*'s (1997) research found psychological abuse to be the most prevalent form noted by carers. The reasons why carers become abusive are multi-varied with possible indications provided by Reay and Browne (2001) who focused upon two distinct situations where individuals were either neglected or abused by their carers. They found significantly higher depression scores present for carers who were abusive whereas there were higher anxiety scores for those who became neglectful. We can also consider the consequences of significant feelings of helplessness and frustration, coupled with the distress from witnessing the suffering of a loved one. An extreme example of this is evidenced by a 77-year-old man who shot and killed his 82-year-old wife who had Alzheimer's disease because he reportedly couldn't stand to see her suffer any more (BBC 2007). Events such as this highlight very forcibly the extreme nature of suffering involved, although it is something that may be largely overlooked as the majority of carers struggle on quietly and *invisibly*, feeling largely unnoticed.

There is a crucial need for carers' needs to be acknowledged and supported. Tabak *et al.*'s (1997) study (see Box 3.3) detailed some of the main stressors involved including the deterioration in a loved one's condition coupled with one's own feelings of being trapped. Some of this is reflected by Cooney and Mortimer (1995) who found that carers who experienced longer periods of care were more prone to feeling socially isolated and becoming physically abusive. Compton *et al.* (1997) linked carers' perception of not receiving help with abuse.

Box 3.3 Causes of anger

The study by Tabak *et al.* (1997) revealed that anger among caregivers derived from three types of stressor:

- Profound mental and behavioural changes in sick loved ones.
- Feelings of physical and mental imprisonment.
- Comparing the present with the rich past and all the dreams and hopes for the future.

The insidious nature of this problem is hard to fully appreciate regarding the steady deterioration in those being cared for, the growing feelings of isolation and stress, as well as an overall lack of support. It is therefore understandable that some end up giving vent to their feelings in desperate ways. One respondent in Boykin and Winland-Brown's (1995: 17) study summed up the dilemma faced in that: 'I get frustrated and take it out on her when she disrupts my sleep and then I feel bad.'

This is the complex and polarized nature of care where carers have conflicting feelings to deal with, as illustrated in the 'causes of anger trap' (see Figure 3.1).

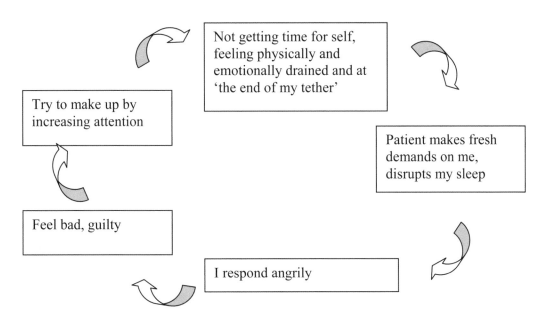

Figure 3.1   The causes of anger trap

Social isolation

Acknowledged in the previous chapter is the sense for the person experiencing dementia of existing in a gradually 'shrinking world'. This can also be applied to the carer, whose own needs and world perspective become progressively restricted in order to focus primarily upon the person they are looking after. There is a strong feeling of *loss* here, incorporating what has already been given up as well as projected future losses in what will now not occur (i.e. goals for retirement). The losses can be summarized as:

- loss of closeness/intimacy;
- loss of socialization;
- loss of future goals.

Loss of closeness/intimacy

A commonly reported issue by carers concerns that of a reduction in intimacy and shared activities with their partner (Betts 2006). Loss of companionship and closeness relates to a feeling of something vital slipping away, indeed the changes can be so profound that carers might describe their partner as 'no longer there' (Murray *et al.* 1999). This type of loss can be felt in different ways as intimacy is powerfully conveyed on a physical as well as emotional level. A much neglected need, especially among the elderly, concerns their sexual needs. It might be due to embarrassment or the expectations that aged people no longer need to satisfy these needs that leads to them being overlooked. The sense of discomfort among healthcare staff can be further heightened where same-sex partners or physical disability are involved, or even where a dementia is HIV/AIDS related. Facilitating intimacy among partners involves looking at one's own feelings and restrictive attitudes as well as the degree of consent that is expressed by both parties. In some cases there may be certain infirmities causing pain or discomfort that need addressing. The Alzheimer's Society (2007) highlight some of the problems for gay carers who are 'forced' to 'come out' to healthcare professionals who have become involved in what was previously a very private relationship. The problem for carers where intimacy needs are not being met is heightened when they seek sexual gratification outside the relationship yet are left with feelings of guilt (Warner 2005). In the television documentary *Malcolm and Barbara*, Barbara recounted feeling very alone: 'I couldn't take a lover before he dies. [Afterwards] if there's any life left in me. I couldn't betray him.' An issue therefore relates to what is done by healthcare staff to address this issue including allowing space for carers to express themselves or making provision within residential care for couples to have time together. Obviously issues of vulnerability and consent would need to be carefully considered and with younger patients there may even be issues of contraceptives to look at.

Perhaps the most striking sense of feeling alone for carers is caused by the progressive distance felt from those who shared their most intimate and treasured memories and experiences. This is indicated by Steele (1994) who states that as shared memories are lost to the other person, carers are left alone with them. It is hard to imagine the depth of distress felt when a partner no longer appreciates or has an awareness of aspects of their life together that once had so much resonance and significance for both partners. In a relationship there are numerous cues that mean a great deal to those involved while at the same time meaning little to others. For example, a song played on the radio, a favourite television programme, a 'magical' holiday destination, a funny recollection or a family joke are all things that can evoke distress and extreme loneliness when having to consider or experience them alone. This is all the more pertinent and painful when applied, for instance, to one's own family, when a partner no longer shares memories of or knows who their children might be. John Bayley's (1998) account of his wife's deterioration and the impact upon their relationship highlights a dual sense of isolation as they became progressively less able to fathom the thoughts and moods of each other.

Loss of socialization

Many people fulfil a large percentage of their socialization needs through contact at work or from individuals they meet when engaged in leisure pursuits. Difficulties are posed for carers therefore when these activities have been given up in order to devote time towards caring for their loved ones. Another factor which causes problems concerns the degree of awkwardness and discomfort felt by former friends and relatives who subsequently find visiting difficult. Comparisons might be drawn with the experience that a number of people have regarding comforting those who are bereaved. Here the choice for many is to maintain a distance, ostensibly to allow others the grieving space it is felt they need, but perhaps also something that is strongly influenced by our own feelings of discomfort and helplessness. Social conventions normally expect that when individuals are ill or encountering difficulties we offer them support and reassurance. This is the presumed position identified by Parsons (1951) with regard to the 'sick role'. However, this process can become exhausted when those we are supporting aren't getting better or have a chronic and longstanding illness. Visits can become progressively less frequent in part through not knowing how to respond but also due to the behaviour and cognitive deterioration exhibited by those with dementia.

Loss of future goals

The previously covered factors address the aspects that have already been lost or are currently being affected. Another significant loss reported by carers relates to what they had planned for the future and what they will not now get to do. This is highlighted by Butcher *et al.* (2001) who report upon the realization that dreams for the golden years of retirement are no longer accessible. The information in Case Study 3.1 shows how carers can struggle with conflicting feelings and where anger and resentment can be directed or felt against their partner.

Case Study 3.1 Arthur

To recap: Arthur is 55 years old, married with three grown-up children and currently has vascular dementia. He previously worked long hours as a local manager for a small transport haulage firm and did not have much time for leisure interests or social activities. Arthur now has poor short-term memory, finds it hard to concentrate and quickly gets confused and angry. He tends now to isolate himself from others.

Arthur

I met with Arthur's wife Marjorie today, who was very tearful and reportedly not coping well. She had written a letter requesting to meet saying how depressed she was feeling, especially when contemplating the future.

'We made so many plans for the future ... all the things we would do together once we both retired. I just feel cheated. I find myself getting very angry with Arthur, especially after all the years I put up with him being absent because of his business. I thought we would travel the world and maybe retire to a cottage by the seaside. That's all just a dream now. I have to remind myself that it's not Arthur's fault although I just get so mad and don't know what to do with these feelings.'

Types of support

In order to meet the support needs of carers and to enable them to maintain what is a physically, psychologically and emotionally draining role, proper help and assistance is needed. It is a role for which many carers have little preparation and those who cope best seem to have support from family, friends and healthcare providers (Karlin *et al.* 2001). There are many problems that carers have to contend with which have a significant impact upon their own state of health. As found by Kerley and Turnbull (1998), isolated and depressed caregivers with little support can develop frustration, despondency and rage resulting in some cases in *giving up syndrome* or even physical and psychological abuse towards those they are caring for.

Activity 3.8

➡ From your present experience and knowledge, what types of support do you think are available to carers?

Carers save the economy £6 billion per year, although the personal cost can be extremely high (Carers UK 2008). It is of paramount importance that practitioners recognize the support needs that carers and family members have and strive to meet these more effectively. Support needs are multi-varied and unique to each carer, incorporating aspects such as respite care, advice and information, financial and social assistance or simply someone to listen. The implications of not properly looking after carers are that numerous physical and mental health needs are created or made worse. Money saved through not attending to carers' welfare is quickly swallowed up as carers present with their own health issues in the future.

Types of support available include:

- respite care;
- advice sheets;
- phone support;
- booklets;
- dementia cafes;
- carers' groups;
- friends and family;
- Telecare;
- online discussion forums.

Advice and support for those experiencing dementia and their carers is available from a range of organizations as diverse as governmental, professional and service-user groups (i.e. the Mental Health Foundation, the Alzheimer's Society and Alzheimer's Disease International). In 2001, the Mental Health Foundation launched a UK-wide service development project entitled the Dementia Advice and Support Service (DASS) which aims to contribute positively to the improvement of services for people with dementia and their families. Projects include 'Lifeline for Carers', a pilot project in Surrey encouraging GP practices to do more to reach out to carers and the South West Surrey Carers Recognition Project which includes regular health checks, more flexible appointment times or home visits, a gateway to other services and counselling and social services referrals. Another initiative is the Alzheimer's Society's online discussion forum Talking Point which helps carers and people with dementia to share their experiences and get advice about coping.

Finding meaning and joy from caring

In contrast to many of the factors highlighted previously, there can be many positive elements encountered by carers through the process of looking after a loved one. Murray *et al.* (1999) highlight some of the positive components of caring as:

- reciprocity for past care and affection;
- desire for continued companionship;
- job satisfaction;
- a perceived unique ability to look after a partner;
- fulfilment of a sense of duty.

In the Murray study of spouses' experience of caring, the onset of illness and growing dependency brought greater emotional closeness for some couples who didn't feel resentful about the personal cost or burden. Some of these issues were linked to a sense of appreciation from their partner and their own personal sense of duty, connected with their marriage vows. As Butcher *et al.* (2001) found, meaning and joy from the caregiver role could be experienced through opportunities to cherish the relationship between caregiver and recipient. The predominant focus was upon enjoying aspects that were still intact and 'making the best of now'. From their results, it was stressed that despite difficulties and hardships (stress, suffering and loss), 78 per cent were able to find positive aspects and meaning in the caregiving process such as cherishing the preciousness of immediate moments. Langner (1995) found that caregivers felt meaning and personal growth accompanied the pain and loss they experienced and that through the act of caregiving they entered a process of rediscovering and redefining themselves as couples.

Some informants in Albinsson and Strang's (2003) study described an increased awareness of the shortness of life which encouraged them to live more intensely in the present. Indeed, in some cases individuals noted that despite all the difficulties and hardships there may be, some very significant benefits were experienced, such as feeling closer. The BBC documentary *George Melly's Last Stand* (BBC4, 7 November 2007) charted the final days in the life of the flamboyant jazz performer as he battled lung cancer and vascular dementia. Shortly before his death, his wife Diana revealed that: 'We've become very good friends again. It's been a progression of getting closer'. Their sense of togetherness and partnership came across very clearly.

In essence, it should not be assumed that the total of the caring experience is negative and it is imperative that healthcare practitioners ensure that carers and those with dementia are properly supported post-diagnosis to savour and maximize the positive elements of their lives together. This entails maintaining a focus on what can still be achieved and enjoyed and not seeing dementia solely in terms of cognitive deterioration and misery (see Best Fit 3.2).

Best Fit 3.2

- Help carers to identify what is positive.
- Help carers to express and verbalize what is difficult.
- Identify practical solutions that can help.
- Maximize opportunities to enjoy and live in the moment.
- Encourage the use of validation approaches which acknowledge the feeling being expressed even where the overall message is incomprehensible.

Moving into residential care

Perhaps the most potent feelings of guilt come when the person with dementia moves into residential care and the passing on of the caregiving role in many cases is done with misgivings and reservations. For many carers this move becomes a necessity and is contemplated when the carer becomes too infirm or the person with dementia's needs become too great to manage. Even when the circumstances make caring at home an unviable option, there can still be strong feelings evoked of abandoning or rejecting the person concerned.

Lundh *et al.*'s (2000) study looked at the predicament facing carers who felt they had no choice other than to place a spouse in a nursing home (see Box 3.4). They highlighted four separate stages fraught with difficult choices and feelings:

1 Making the decision.
2 Making the move.
3 Adjusting to the move.
4 Reorientation.

The Lundh study found relatively little planning or prior discussion about the move to a care home being carried out with those concerned.

Activity 3.9

Consider the issues facing carers when choosing residential care with regards the various stages of:

→ Making the decision.
→ Making the move.
→ Adjusting to the move.
→ Reorientation.

Box 3.4 The carer's experience of placing a partner in residential care

Making the decision – the placement decision was not the result of an acute health crisis but rather a growing awareness of their inability to carry on in a caring role. Despite legitimation, spouses still felt they had let their partner down, seeing it as a form of treachery. In a number of cases the move was not discussed with spouses and carers reached the decision in isolation or through minimal contact with health agencies.

Making the move – a prevailing feeling among carers was of powerlessness and emptiness. After suggesting a move, professionals usually played a minor role leaving the family to cope emotionally and practically. Some coped by immersing themselves in the practicalities of the move although found evenings hardest. Moving from hospital was less traumatic than moving from home, with the first stage of separation already occurring.

Adjusting to the move – the period immediately following the move was found to be the hardest. Initial feelings of freedom and relief from the physical burden of care were countered by feelings of guilt, powerlessness and the sense of being an 'outsider' in their partner's care. They found it hard to influence care and did not feel that staff were listening to their suggestions.

Reorientation – most respondents felt it important to maintain contact with their spouse, such as through bringing the daily paper and sharing news with them. They also faced the difficulty and apprehension of trying to renew contacts in the community.

Adapted from Lundh *et al.* (2000)

Nolan and Dellasega's (1999) study shows some of the mixed feelings when placing a relative in residential care with emotions as opposing as relief and guilt. Feelings that one is betraying and letting one's partner down are present even when the role of carer has become intolerable. Armstrong (2000) covers some of the reasons why individuals could not care for relatives at home any more:

- incontinence;
- sheer physical dependency (i.e. lifting);
- wandering;
- verbal and physical aggression.

Ryan and Scullion (2000) reflect the findings that admission to a nursing home might be held off for as long as possible but deteriorating health for carers and those they are caring for left them with no other option. There is also a strong desire to protect the individual and prevent them getting harmed, something that might occur due to their current environment and the strain upon the carer. For example, Kellett

(1999) reports that carers at times have to lock relatives in the house when doing simple activities. A strong illustration of this experience for those with dementia is provided by Bernlef's (1988) *Out of Mind*, a fictional first-person account of the dementing process:

> *Hunting for things. If there's anything I detest that's it. Where are my keys? And what imbecile has locked all the doors? Robert follows me like a good dog as I try the kitchen door, the laundry-room door and the outside door. Vera must have double-locked it. How could she be so silly? ... On the shelf in the laundry room I find what I am looking for at once. I take a screwdriver and hammer from the wooden toolbox and go to the door. It is easier than I expected. I wedge the screwdriver between the door and the post. After a few hammer blows the door leaps open towards me. Robert slips out immediately and barks, relieved that he too has been freed from his imprisonment.*
>
> (Bernlef 1988: 32)

This is a powerful account which highlight the 'plight' of the person with dementia who subsequently feels trapped and uncertain as to why a simple wish such as going out for a walk can't be fulfilled. It is something which can provide carers with a dilemma if wishing for example to go and post a letter or go to the corner shop to buy a pint of milk but not feeling like going through the arduous process each time of preparing a partner for the outing.

Advice about the move into residential care is given by dementia support organizations such as Alzheimer's Disease International (2004):

> *The decision to move someone you care about or love into a nursing home is a difficult and painful decision to make. Yet caring for someone with dementia can become a 24-hour occupation and there comes a time when short breaks of respite care will not provide sufficient relief. Eventually, you risk damaging your own health if you do not consider moving the person to a home, where they can get the 24-hour help they need.*

This painful and difficult process is vividly highlighted in a number of biographical accounts including *Remind Me Who I Am Again Please* by Linda Grant (1999) concerning the guilt felt over her mother Rose's move into residential care. Guilt is also a strong feature in Michael Ignatieff's (1993) *Scar Tissue* with a poignant passage illustrating how his brother travelled across a number of states to accompany him and in a sense share out the degree of guilt felt as their mother went into care. These examples illustrate the need to properly support family and carers during this traumatic process as well as to involve them fully in the planning process. The negative public image of care homes, however, generally means that a move into residential care is seen as a last resort and consequently impinges upon the level of involvement or preparation prior to the move (Lundh *et al.* 2000). As Cotter *et al.* (1998) indicate there is frequently little discussion with the person or their carer even when the need becomes apparent, making the move something that is dominated by professionals.

Case Study 3.2 Elsie

To recap: Elsie is an 83-year-old woman currently living in a residential care setting. She is a widower and has two children and eight grandchildren. She previously worked as a veterinarian, had an active social life, was keen on outdoor activities and stimulated herself with word puzzles and crosswords. Her cognition has steadily deteriorated as has her confidence and motivation for activities. Her family now seldom visit her.

Elsie

I met with Elsie's family today and was struck by how difficult they have found her moving into residential care. In particular, one of her granddaughters told me that she felt very bad about being unable to help and feels partly to blame for her grandmother not being able to remain in her own home. She lives two hours' drive away and is a single mother with two young children. She has a part-time job and says that she feels exhausted and stressed tying to help, although cannot do any more. It does not, as she told me, stop her feeling incredibly guilty and very sad.

As well as partners, the experience for others in the family can be equally as significant and distressing (see Case Study 3.2). Other family roles bring with them their own specific expectations, for example where children are having to care for elderly and infirm parents. There is the socially recognized or personally felt obligation to pay one's parent back for early care. A situation where one can never do enough is tailor-made for feelings of guilt (Samuelsson *et al.* 2001).

Activity 3.10

Have a look at *A Positive Choice – Choosing Long-Stay Care for a Person with Dementia* (Alzheimer's Scotland 2007):

➡ www.alzscot.org/downloads/positivechoice.pdf

Partnerships

A major issue for carers once relatives have entered residential care relates to feelings of exclusion. Many carers have a wish to maintain some level of input in order to support their relelative as well as to feel needed (Armstrong 2001). Effective partnerships are therefore vital with continuity being provided for both parties and potential benefits for all individuals concerned. Nolan and Dellasega (1999) state that staff should create a welcoming environment that supports and encourages carers to become involved if desired. For partnerships to work effectively there should be reciprocity as healthcare staff also have needs to be acknowledged, such as relatives/ carers not having unrealistic expectations of them as well as recognizing and appreciating what they are doing. A need here is to acquaint carers of certain constraints and to foster effective ongoing communication channels. The carer's role in ongoing care cannot be overestimated as we have here the custodian of the person's life experiences. It is someone who is ideally placed to act as an advocate and adviser to care staff. Activity 3.11 provides you with an opportunity to consider maintaining partnership approaches between healthcare staff and carers, and practice recommendations are provided in Best Fit 3.3.

Activity 3.11

➡ How are partnerships between carers and healthcare staff best maintained in practice?

What do you feel the benefits are for:	*What might the potential difficulties be for:*
The carer	The carer
The patient	The patient
The staff	The staff

Best Fit 3.3

- Develop partnership approaches with carers whenever possible.
- Promote opportunities for carers to maintain as active a caring role as possible.
- Provide opportunities for support and supervision for carers.
- Look into insurance and risk aspects with regards to enabling carers to get involved.

Facing the end

In a study conducted by Keene *et al.* (2001) the immediate causes of death for those with dementia were pneumonia, cardiovascular disease and pulmonary embolus. Over half of those in the study group died in a debilitated state due to severe dementia, being incontinent, unable to walk and having severe difficulties in communicating.

Clearly, it is a time of great sadness and difficulty for carers as they prepare for the inevitable loss and start to contemplate their life for the years ahead.

Activity 3.12

➡ What do you think the carer's feelings might be when those they have been caring for die?
➡ What difficulties might they face when trying to re-establish their own lives?

Activity 3.12 asks you to look at the period following a partner's death and the difficulty in trying to rebuild one's life. Clearly, feelings and experiences will vary from person to person, influenced by the nature of their relationship and the severity and length of the caring process. The person's death can evoke strongly conflicting feelings, polarized between sadness and relief. It might be presumed that carers who have had a particularly hard and drawn-out process would feel relieved, yet as Steele (1994) outlines, caring has in a sense filled that person's entire focus and the grieving can be very intense.

As Schulz *et al.* (2006) indicate, most family carers adapt well to the death of their relative although a sizeable number (20 per cent) experience complicated grief and depression. Those suffering the most had depressive symptoms prior to the person's death, and were caring for more cognitively impaired individuals. Interventions aimed at reducing depression and the sense of burden experienced were effective concerning the subsequent emergence of psychiatric morbidity.

Another core factor concerning the way that carers cope with bereavement is the level of support experienced and the possibility of continued help from family and friends (Almberg *et al.* 2000). In Hebert *et al.*'s (2006) study, a proportion (23 per cent) of caregivers were not prepared for the death of their loved one and experienced more anxiety and complicated grief. Tweedy and Guarnaccia's (2008) research illustrated some gender differences in the grieving process, with bereaved husbands showing a decrease in depression over time yet wives continuing to report increased depression.

As well as grieving for their deceased relative, many carers subsequently struggle to re-establish their lives and regain social contacts and leisure interests. The time and space now available to them may seem like a void, characterized by profound feelings of sadness and loneliness. For some, the process of caring had provided them with a sense of purpose and of feeling needed and they subsequently have to find other ways to fulfil these needs. The difficulties for carers in restarting their lives may relate to:

- present age;
- health state;
- confidence;
- relationships that have become strained.

These issues will place a significant pressure upon carers when attempting to rebuild previously established relationships. As Costello and Kendrick (2000) indicate, there may also be difficulties in starting new relationships with an emotional bond with the deceased partner being retained. Clearly, this can be an intensely complex and distressing process, particularly if unresolved or difficult issues present for those concerned. It shows that proper support is needed even though the person's death had been expected. Space to ventilate, discuss and work through emotions is needed (see Best Fit 3.4 for further recommendations).

Best Fit 3.4

- Promote opportunities for carers to express their feelings about their bereavement.
- Look into providing contact with/support from others undergoing similar experiences.

Conclusion

This chapter has identified some real issues facing carers of individuals with dementia. As stated, their experience needn't necessarily be all negative and some carers can experience some very meaningful and important moments with their family member post-diagnosis. This might provide the impetus to focus upon and savour what they still have of their life together where a diagnosis is not regarded as a death sentence. However, the enormous strain and burden endured by many carers who are left to cope with immensely difficult and arduous care must be acknowledged. This involves the totality of their experience where the strain can be emotional, social, psychological and physical. As the number of those with dementia continues to rise, so does the number of carers. Their support needs have to be taken seriously as otherwise the outcome will be larger numbers of people presenting with 'new' healthcare needs as a consequence of their unremitting and incredibly taxing caring role.

Key points

- Healthcare professionals need to be cognizant of the nature of the carer's 'burden' in terms of physical, psychological and social stressors.
- A move into residential care should be done through a partnership approach (person with dementia, carers, family, friends and healthcare staff).
- Carers need proper support and respite. They also need opportunities to express and work through their feelings.
- It should be recognized that the grieving process for many carers begins before the death of their partner. Help and space to better understand and deal with this experience is needed.
- The carer should be given opportunities to maintain involvement in care even after a move into residential care.

References

Albinsson, L. and Strang, P. (2003) Existential concerns of families of late-stage dementia patients: questions of freedom, choices, isolation, death and meaning, *Journal of Palliative Medicine*, 6(2): 225–35.

Almberg, B., Grafstrom, M. and Winblad, B. (2000) Caregivers of relatives with dementia: experiences encompassing social support and bereavement, *Aging and Mental Health*, 4(1): 82–9.

Alzheimer's Disease International (2004) *Getting Help*, www.alz.co.uk/carers/help.html#homes, accessed 11 December 2007.

Alzheimer's Society (2007) *What is the Lesbian, Gay, Bisexual and Transgender Carers group?*, www.alzheimers.org.uk/site/scripts/documents_info.php?categoryID=200204&documentID=322, accessed 27 February 2008.

Alzheimer's Society (2008) *Dealing with Guilt*, www.alzheimers.org.uk/factsheet/516Factsheet guilty, accessed 3 April 2009.

Anderson, R. (1987) The unremitting burden on carers, *British Medical Journal*, 204: 73.

Archbold, P. and Stewart, B. (1996) The nature of the family caregiving role and nursing interventions for caregiving families, in E. Swanson and T. Tripp-Reimer (eds) *Advances in Gerontological Nursing: Issues for the 21st Century*. New York: Springer Publishing.

Armstrong, M. (2000) Factors affecting the decision to place a relative with dementia into residential care, *Nursing Standard*, 14(16): 33–7.

Armstrong, M. (2001) The pressures felt by informal carers of people with dementia, *Nursing Standard*, 15(17): 47–55.

Bayley, J. (1998) *Iris: A Memoir of Iris Murdoch*. London: Abacus.

BBC (2007) Italian shoots wife in hospital, http://news.bbc.co.uk/1/hi/world/europe/7123460.stm, accessed 3 December 2007.

Bernlef, J. (1988) *Out of Mind*. London: Faber & Faber.

Betts, K. (2006) The transition to caregiving: the experience of family members embarking on the dementia caregiving career, *Journal of Gerontological Social Work*, 47(3/4): 3–29.

Boykin, A. and Winland-Brown, J. (1995) The dark side of caregiving: challenges of caregiving, *Journal of Gerontological Nursing*, 21(5): 13–19.

Brodaty, H., Green, A. and Low, L. (2005) Family carers for people with dementia, in A. Burns, J. O'Brien and D. Ames (eds) *Dementia*, 3rd edn. London: Hodder Arnold.

Butcher, H., Holkup, P. and Buckwalter, K. (2001) The experience of caring for a family member with Alzheimer's disease, *Western Journal of Nursing Research*, 23(1): 33–55.

Carers UK (2008) *Facts about Caring*, ww.carersuk.org/Home, accessed 1 April 2009.

Compton, S., Flanagan, P. and Gregg, W. (1997) Elder abuse in people with dementia in Northern Ireland: prevalence and predictors in cases referred to a psychiatry of old age service, *International Journal of Geriatric Psychiatry*, 12(6): 632–5.

Cooney, M. and Mortimer, A. (1995) Elder abuse and dementia: a pilot study, *International Journal of Social Psychiatry*, 41(4): 276–83.

Coope, B., Ballard, C., Saad, K., Patel, A., Bentham, P., Bannister, C., Graham, C. and Wilcock, G. (1995) The prevalence of depression in the carers of dementia sufferers, *International Journal of Geriatric Psychiatry*, 10: 237–42.

Costello, J. and Kendrick, K. (2000) Grief and older people: the making or breaking of emotional bonds following partner loss in later life, *Journal of Advanced Nursing*, 32(6): 1374–82.

Cotter, A., Meyer, J. and Roberts, S. (1998) Humanity or bureaucracy: the transition from hospital to long term residential care, *Nursing Times Research*, 3: 247–56.

Eisdorfer, C. (1991) Caregiving: an emerging risk factor for emotional and physical pathology, *Bulletin of the Menninger Clinic*, 55: 238–47.

Gallagher, D., Rose, J., Rivera, P., Lovett, S. and Thompson, L. (1989) Prevalence of depression in family caregivers, *The Gerontologist*, 29: 449–56.

Grant, L. (1999) *Remind Me who I am Again Please*. London: Granta.

Hebert , R., Dang, Q. and Schultz, R. (2006) Preparedness for the death of a loved one and mental health in bereaved caregivers of patients with dementia: findings from the REACH study, *Journal of Palliative Medicine*, 9(3): 683–93.

Ignatieff, M. (1993) *Scar Tissue*. London: Viking.

Karlin, N., Bell, P. and Noah, J. (2001) Long-term consequences of the Alzheimer's caregiver role: a qualitative analysis, *American Journal of Alzheimer's Disease and other Dementias*, 16(3): 177–82.

Keene, J., Hope, T., Fairburn, C. and Jacoby, R. (2001) Death and dementia, *International Journal of Geriatric Psychiatry*, 16(10): 969–74.

Kellett, U. (1999) Transition in care: family carer's experience of nursing home placement, *Journal of Advanced Nursing*, 29(6): 1474–81.

Kerley, L. and Turnbull, J. (1998) Stress in caregivers, in R. Hamdy, J. Turnbull, J. Edwards and M. Lancaster (eds) *Alzheimer's Disease: A Handbook for Caregivers*, 3rd edn. St Louis, MO: Mosby.

Kjellin, L. and Östman, M. (2005) Relatives of psychiatric inpatients: do physical violence and suicide attempts of patients influence family burden and participation in care? *Nordic Journal of Psychiatry*, 59: 7–11.

Kurrie, S., Sadler, P., Lockwood, K. and Cameron, I. (1997) Elder abuse: prevalence, intervention and outcomes in patients referred to four aged care assessment teams, *Medical Journal of Australia*, 166(3): 119–22.

Langner, S. (1995) Finding meaning in caring for elderly relatives: loss and personal growth, *Holistic Nursing Practice*, 9(3): 75–84.

Lundh, U., Sandberg, J. and Nolan, M. (2000) 'I don't have any other choice': spouses' experiences of placing a partner in a care home for older people in Sweden, *Journal of Advanced Nursing*, 32(5): 1178–86.

Mace, N. (1992) *The 36 Hour Day: A Family Guide to Caring at Home for People with Alzheimer's Disease and Other Confusional Illnesses*. London: Hodder & Stoughton.

Mittelman, M., Ferris, S., Shulman, E., Steinberg, G., Ambinder, A., Mackell, J. and Cohen, J. (1995) A comprehensive support group program: effect on depression in spouse-caregivers of AD patients, *The Gerontologist*, 35: 792–802.

Murray, J., Schneider, J., Banerjee, S. and Mann, A. (1999) Eurocare; a cross-national study of co-resident spouse carers for people with Alzheimer's disease: ii – a qualitative analysis of the experience of caregiving, *International Journal of Geriatric Psychiatry*, 14: 662–7.

Nolan, M. and Dellasega, C. (1999) 'It's not the same as him being at home': creating caring partnerships following nursing home placement, *Journal of Clinical Nursing*, 8(6): 723–30.

Parsons, T. (1951) *The Social System*. Glencoe, IL: Free Press.

Reay, A. and Browne, K. (2001) Risk factor characteristics in carers who physically abuse or neglect their elderly dependants, *Aging and Mental Health*, 5(1): 56–62.

Ryan, A. and Scullion, H. (2000) Nursing home placement: an exploration of the experiences of family carers, *Journal of Advanced Nursing*, 32(5): 1187–95.

Samuelsson, A., Annerstedt, L., Elmståhl, S., Samuelsson, S. and Grafström, M. (2001) Burden of responsibility experienced by family caregivers of elderly dementia sufferers, *Scandinavian Journal of Caring Science*, 15: 25–33.

Schulz, R. and Beach, S. (1999) Caregiving as a risk factor for mortality: the caregiver health effects study, *Journal of the American Medical Association*, 282: 2215–19.

Schulz, R., Boerner, K., Shear, K. and Gitlin, N. (2006) Predictors of complicated grief among dementia caregivers: a prospective study of bereavement, *American Journal of Geriatric Psychiatry*, 14(8): 650–8.

Schulze, B. and Rössler, W. (2005) Caregiver burden in mental illness: review of measurement, findings and interventions in 2004–2005, *Current Opinion in Psychiatry*, 18(6): 684–91.

Steele, C. (1994) Management of the family, in A. Burns and R. Levy (eds) *Dementia*. London: Arnold.

Stevenson, R. (2007) So near and yet so far away, *Metro*, 23 January.

Tabak, N., Ehrenfeld, M. and Alpert, R. (1997) Feelings of anger among caregivers of patients with Alzheimer's disease, *International Journal of Nursing Practice*, 3(2): 84–8.

Tweedy, M. and Guarnaccia, C. (2008) Change in depression of spousal caregivers of dementia patients following patient's death, *Omega: Journal of Death and Dying*, 56(3): 217–28.

Vassilas, C. (2003) Dementia and literature, *Advances in Psychiatric Treatment*, 9: 439–45.

Warner, J. (2005) Sexuality and dementia, in A. Burns, J. O'Brien and D. Ames (eds) *Dementia*, 3rd edn. London: Hodder Arnold.

Further reading

Alzheimer's Scotland (2007) *A Positive Choice – Choosing Long Stay Care for a Person with Dementia*, www.alzscot.org/downloads/positivechoice.pdf, accessed 10 January 2008.

Alzheimer's Society (2006) *Caring for Someone with Dementia*, www.alzheimers.org.uk/Caring_for_someone_with_dementia/Coping_with_caring/info_guilt.htm, accessed 11 May 2006.

English National Board (1999) *Learning from Each Other: The Involvement of People Who Use Services and Their Carers in Education*. London: ENB.

Mental Health Foundation (2001) *First Signs*, www.mentalhealth.org.uk/publications/?EntryId5=38689, accessed 20 March 2009.

Lindgren, C., Connelly, C. and Gaspar, H. (1999) Grief in spouse and children caregivers of dementia patients, *Western Journal of Nursing Research*, 21(4): 521–37.

4 Attitudes

Objectives: After reading this chapter you should be able to:

➡ Discuss how stigmatizing views and age discriminatory beliefs are established.
➡ Explore how self-awareness can increase our understanding of how we think about the person with dementia.
➡ Reflect upon the factors which influence how we engage with the person experiencing dementia.

Clinical problems (the practitioner's perspective)

'As people age they become less able to look after themselves.'

'We don't have time to wait for Elsie to dress herself before breakfast and so need to do it for her.'

'I know he prefers to be known as Charles but we all call him Charley.'

'The nature of dementia means that people will only get worse and so need to be looked after.'

And yet ... these commonly held attitudes and discriminatory beliefs foster a paternalistic culture which in turn promotes dependent and hopelessness behaviours.

Introduction

This chapter is concerned with attitudes and the ways in which personal beliefs and societal influences help to shape the responses we make to others. The main focus is upon our feelings and resultant attitudes towards people as a consequence of two core themes: their age and the presence of dementia. This brings in the notion of *double discrimination*, where individuals are stigmatized because of the discriminatory views that are held about older people *and* those with mental health problems – in this instance, dementia. It is generally the case that low expectations are held about individuals in relation to both of these categories.

Figure 4.1 considers a series of factors, by no means exhaustive, that can influence the ways a person with dementia is perceived. At the base is the concept of double

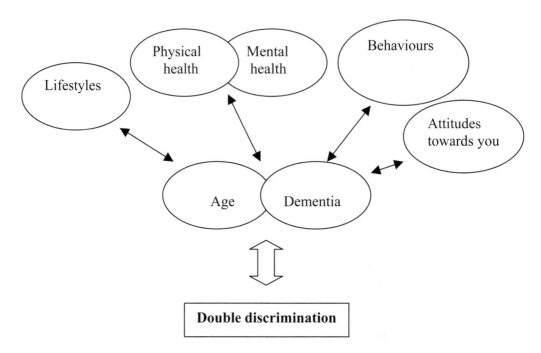

Figure 4.1   Double discrimination

discrimination where personal attitudes are generated by beliefs and views that are held about a person by virtue of their age and condition of dementia. These beliefs and views incorporate opinions about a person's physical and mental health state as well as their displayed behaviours and lifestyle choices, while also being mindful of the attitudes they communicate.

The notion of double discrimination does not account for all the other potential reasons a person may encounter prejudicial treatment. The multi-factorial nature of dementia means that it may affect people who already live with severe mental health problems, such as schizophrenia or bipolar disorder, as well as those who develop anxiety and depression as a consequence of their failing cognition. They might also encounter societal prejudice or personal bigotry because of disability, sexual orientation, cultural practices or religious beliefs.

This notion of double discrimination towards the older person, how they live with their dementia and assumptions about their competence (and *compos mentis*) may explain why low expectations can be held about them. It should be noted here that not all individuals with dementia are older adults, as according to the Alzheimer's Society (2007), 2.2 per cent of people with dementia in the UK are those with younger-onset dementia. We can include within this group those with HIV, the most common cause of dementia in people under the age of 40 years, occurring in the same regions of the brain as Parkinson's disease and Huntington's disease. AIDS dementia is one of 70 chronological conditions that occur in people with HIV/AIDS (Brew 2001). Discrimination also applies to people with Down's syndrome who have been identified as becoming particularly vulnerable to developing Alzheimer's disease, affecting at least 9 per cent of people aged 40 to 49 years, 36 per cent of people aged 50 to 59 years and 54 per cent of people aged 60 to 69 years (Turk *et al.* 2001). While the younger-onset group does include a significant amount of people, estimated at approximately 15,000 currently in the UK (Alzheimer's Society 2007), the main focus of this chapter is upon attitudinal responses and feelings regarding the components of old age and dementia.

Working in practice

Our understanding and feelings about older people who experience dementia will be developed through a range of experiences including previous clinical practice. The subsequent beliefs and values fostered will in part be related to the ways in which the caring milieu was perceived and implemented, the types of interventions employed and the clinical activities undertaken. You might have worked in practice areas where person-centred approaches are actively encouraged and there is a general air of optimism, or alternatively in settings where a general air of pessimism pervades and little more than physical needs are catered for. The learning taken away from practice allied with what we get from the media, peers or through family experience plays a significant part in shaping our overall feelings about dementia care. We have observed that healthcare students about to commence their dementia care placements varied significantly in their attitudinal views and levels of enthusiasm. The feelings and expectations about entering a new clinical environment are reflected in Exercise 1 (full details are provided in Chapter 9).

Exercise 1: Circle of concerns

This exercise encouraged healthcare students to explore their attitudes and feelings towards older people with dementia prior to them commencing placements within community, daycare and residential settings. The focus was upon particular apprehensions held about working within dementia care and predicted difficulties in meeting individual wants and needs. Doubts and concerns appeared to be influenced by a variety of factors including:

- the student's age (most of them were in their early twenties);
- prior negative care experiences;
- lack of experience.

The students were asked to write about a concern they had about working with individuals experiencing dementia and these accounts were then randomly distributed to other group members. Concerns were then aired in the group, with positive coping strategies contemplated. The tenor of these group discussions was maintained as optimistic with emphasis upon what could be done to make a difference to the individual with dementia. Some of the examples of healthcare students' concerns (in italics) are included below with a range of responses from fellow students.

- *Not being able to carry out an aspect of care.* This needn't necessarily be seen as a failing on the student's part. The importance here is in having the opportunity to discuss the issue with colleagues and understand the nature of the problem as well as alternative ways of intervening.
- *Dealing with difficult or challenging situations.* The importance here is in appreciating what the term 'challenging' actually means and the 'difficulty' not being regarded as solely located in the person with dementia but also located in part with the carer and the person's environment. Challenging behaviour was also considered to reflect an attempt at communicating particular needs which were not being met or comprehended.
- *Having difficulty with communication.* Words can be regarded as simply one way of communicating. If this is ineffective the appropriate use of non-verbal behaviours (i.e. touch, eye contact, facial expressions) can provide the necessary interpersonal skills to promote engagement. Silence and attending (use of personal space) can also provide comfort without the obligation to talk.
- *Not being able to deal with aggressive behaviours.* Dealing with aggressive behaviour involves being able to maintain personal safety as well as a safe environment. It is also important to understand possible antecedents and contributory factors. Another way of looking at situations is to reframe aggressive incidents – for example, regarding the person as frightened, helpless or frustrated.
- *Discomfort at dealing with personal care (including incontinence).* Our discomfort in being involved with somebody's intimate personal care may be negligible compared with the sense of embarrassment or shame felt by the person who has been incontinent or is unable to manage their own hygiene and self-care needs.
- *Being able to make a difference.* The need here is to focus upon achievable goals or the significance of interventions to those concerned. What might be a very small issue for us could be massively significant for the person with dementia. For example, a briefly shared pleasant moment can have a huge impact and resonance upon another's sense of well-being.

The importance of this exercise was in finding a starting point for students to contemplate their forthcoming clinical placements and to freely express their concerns and anticipated difficulties. Group members were very supportive of each other's concerns and contributions were both thoughtful and constructive. What did emerge strongly was that many of these concerns were based upon assumptions and stereotypical notions of those who are elderly or individuals who are experiencing problems with dementia. A number of misapprehensions were quickly countered by students who had significant prior experience of working within dementia care.

What are attitudes?

Attitudes provide us with a way of organizing our beliefs, feelings and behaviours so that we can arrive at an evaluation towards a person or an issue. The word 'attitude' has its origins in the Latin word *aptus*, which means 'fit and ready for action'. This ancient interpretation referred to something that could have been directly observed, such as athletes in a sporting event. In contemporary times, attitudes can be viewed more as a construct that, although not directly observed, precedes a person's behaviours and guides how they make choices and decisions concerning their subsequent actions. Attitudes that we form could be described as relatively stable feelings and govern the extent to which a given event might be evaluated in a positive or negative way. There is not always a clear association between the behaviours we exhibit and the attitudes we hold, although each clearly has an influence on the other. An earlier view was of a tripartite model (Rosenberg and Hovland 1960) that incorporated the following components:

- *affective* (personal feelings and emotions – what we like or dislike);
- *behavioural* (intentions or action tendencies);
- *cognitive* (opinions and beliefs).

These components were thought to be dynamic, in that each could influence and become influenced by being presented with new or different information. This describes an attitude as a particular evaluation of an object that could influence emotions, knowledge or behaviour in regard to that object. As a generalization, we tend to have positive attitudes towards attitude objects that are consistent with the goals we have, but may develop negative attitudes towards attitude objects that we feel are likely to cause us frustration or prevent our needs being met. Fishbein and Ajzen (1975) have argued that attitudes are learned predispositions that respond in a consistently favourable or unfavourable way towards a given object, person or event and include certain factors:

- people are not born with attitudes, they learn them through experience;
- attitudes tend to be stable and relatively enduring;
- attitudes are a means by which people make judgements in either a positive or negative way.

The attitudes we form towards other people are influenced in part by the impressions (fleeting or lasting) that they create and we may evaluate these as being distinguishing qualities or characteristics of that person.

Activity 4.1

Consider your family, friends and colleagues	Consider people in the public eye (e.g. celebrities, politicians)
⇩	⇩

What is it that you like about them?

☐	☐
☐	☐
☐	☐
☐	☐

From your lists of attributes, what personal attraction comparisons can you make?

How we seek to construct our attitudes is in part based upon our life experiences, the influence that other people have had on us and our emotional reaction to particular situations. The formation of an attitude from direct experience allows us to arrive at either a positive or negative evaluation about that event. For example, going to the dentist for some people may engender past childhood memories whereby lasting impressions of sights, sounds and smells influence their current attitudes. Furthermore, if there are associations with painful memories, entering the surgery and being greeted by dental aromas may rekindle feelings of uncertainty and reinforce certain behaviours. We are not intending to malign the dental profession and its inclusion is but an example of how childhood experiences can remain in adulthood. We can also consider the extent to which childhood attendance in any healthcare setting (as a patient in hospital or visiting an accident and emergency unit) could have a profound influence on adult attitudes when revisiting hospitals. When direct experiences are especially negative and distressing our beliefs can become more salient than others, a view reflected by Oskamp (1977) who argues that traumatic and frightening experiences can be important in the formation of attitudes. Attitudes can also be formed through observation where there are no direct reinforcers present. Bandura (1973) views this as *learning by observation*, where there is the tendency for a person to reproduce the actions, attitudes and emotional responses exhibited by others.

Activity 4.2

➡ In what ways do you formulate attitudes towards a person or group of people?

Activity 4.2 asks you to think about your attitudes towards other people. The identifying of certain commonalities may go some way in determining how we formulate attitudes towards a person or group of people. Below is a less than exhaustive list that we are sure you could add to.

- *Age groups* – adolescents, middle-aged and older people.
- *Lifestyles* – thrill-seeking behaviours or a sedentary existence.
- *Occupations* – student, high-achieving professional, long-term unemployed.
- *Behaviours* – hostile, self-abusive, addictive or caring.
- *Language used* – difficult to understand, confused or incoherent.
- *Illness* – contracted by self-indulgence or unexplainable, treatable or not.
- *Media reporting* – of human vulnerabilities and erratic or difficult to explain behaviours towards oneself or other people.

Any of the factors outlined above could have an impact upon the judgemental interpretations we make about people, their lifestyle and present demeanour. Figure 4.2 considers how attitudes could be formed and some of these determinants include societal values, media commentaries, individual behaviours and appearances. A second contributing factor, namely 'roots of discontent', can promote more rigid and judgemental attitudes.

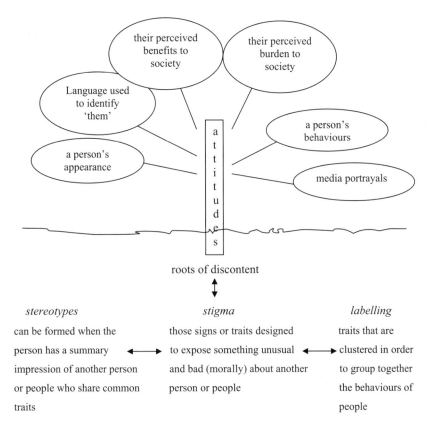

Figure 4.2 The attitudes tree

'Roots of discontent' can be fed by the ways in which stigmatizing attitudes are developed, something which contributes to the stereotyping and labelling processes. The entrenchment of negative attitudes is reinforced by the language (often pejorative) used to describe the *object person*, where their perceived productivity and value to society creates an impression of either benefit or burden. Further detrimental processes are created by negatively perceived behaviour and appearance, which along with visual and narrative messages conveyed through varied media products, provide a prescriptive interpretation or label.

The following sections outline some of the core aspects related to attitude formation, and address stereotypes, stigma and labelling.

Stereotypes

- First described scientifically by Lippman (1922), stereotypes were treated as simplified mental images that acted as templates to help interpret the huge diversity of the social world.
- Stereotypical attitudes are generalizations about a person or a group of people that often have a prejudicial component. We can develop stereotypes when we are unwilling or unable to obtain all the necessary information that will allow for a fair judgement about a situation or people. Sometimes in the absence of 'all the information', stereotypes allow us to 'fill in the gaps'.
- The need for stereotypes can be seen as a way of helping us to make sense of the overwhelming amount of information that we are exposed to on a daily basis. We cope with this by classifying data and grouping it according to familiar patterns.
- The establishment of stereotypes may lead to a variety of interpretations that are usually basic images, often derogatory, which when applied to groups of people create visible differences and can become central aspects of prejudice and discrimination.
- Societal institutionalization provided the structure necessary to form stereotypes about elderly people and encourage prejudicial behaviours (Bond 1992).

Stigma

- The word 'stigma' has its origins in Greek slaves, who had a mark or brand placed on them as a way of distinguishing and separating them from free men.
- Goffman (1963: 1) defined stigma as something undesirable; 'a trait deeply discrediting' with attributes that 'disqualify one from full social acceptance'. His research interests had a focus on psychiatric stigma, however he did comment that the differences between a normal and stigmatized person were a question of perspective, not reality, and that stigma is in the 'eye of the beholder'.
- Stigmatization occurs when a person possesses (or is believed to possess) 'some attribute or characteristic that conveys a sound identity that is devalued in a particular social context' (Crocker *et al.* 1998: 505).

- Stigma exists when labelling, negative stereotyping, exclusion, discrimination and low social status co-occur in a power situation that allows these processes to unfold (Link and Phelan 2001).

Labelling

- In the nineteenth century the medical community began to preface various physical conditions with the term 'senile' to link diseases to elderly individuals. Following the institution of old age pension programmes, individuals of 65 years and older were categorized into one homogenous group.
- Labelling influences the ways in which a person or a group of people are perceived. Cohen (1982) argues that one's identity and views of self are created primarily as a result of how others act and respond towards us.

Ageism

In principle, *ageism* refers to the stereotyping of or discrimination against any group based upon their age. As we become older our subjective notions of young and old may well change with the passage of time. Butler (1969) coined the term ageism to describe a form of bigotry, similar to racism and sexism, with respect to age and believed it would parallel if not replace racism as the prominent issue of the future. He defined ageism as prejudice by one age group towards other age groups and suggested it was based on 'a personal revulsion to and distaste for growing old, disease, disability: and a fear of powerlessness, "usefulness" and death' (1969: 243). This sentiment seems geared more towards discrimination about old age, although negative attitudinal views can work both ways with both groups (old and young) viewing the other as a completely different and somewhat distasteful species.

Attitudes towards younger people

While specific attitudinal beliefs are held about older people it is interesting to consider the reverse dynamic – the ways in which young people/adolescents are regarded (see Activity 4.3). As each subsequent generation emerges out of childhood, they create their own sense of identity (appearance, behaviour and language) along with distinct attitudes and perceptions to lifestyle issues and world events. To some degree this makes them unfathomable to older generations who struggle to comprehend their world perspective.

Activity 4.3

Complete the sentences below.

➡ 'My attitudes towards young people/adolescents are … '
➡ 'These values suggest … '

The age you are and your particular life experiences will influence the types of attitudes you express about younger people. For example, you may be chronologically young (or have a youthful outlook on life), have experienced a nurturing role (i.e. as a parent or grandparent), had direct contact with positive or negative youth behaviours or have been influenced by media messages about young people in our society. Each generation has spawned its own youth culture, allowing young people to promote their own 'unique' and often 'uniformed' appearance while also adopting a language that represents their understanding of self, others and their world. This provides a statement about their beliefs, values and attitudes, and makes them visually stand out from other groups within society. Since the middle of the last century it would appear to have become the choice of each generation to express their difference by establishing youth movements, such as beatniks, Teddy boys, mods and rockers, hippies, skinheads, punks, new romantics, goths and chavs, to name but a few. All of this is geared towards the younger generation distancing themselves from the older generations whom they regard as different from themselves. It reflects the underlying sentiment within ageism where the worth of older people is denigrated, and as Butler (1987: 22) reflects: 'they suddenly cease to identify with their elders as human beings ... at times ageing becomes an expedient method by which society promotes viewpoints about the aged in order to relieve itself from responsibility towards them'. Perhaps the first line of Butler's quote also reflects some of the societal views about adolescents, fuelled in no small part by media reporting. This regards younger people as 'hoodies', 'yobs' or 'layabouts', all resulting in a wide divide being created between these two very disparate age groups. One point of note here is a consideration of the potentially negative attitude that some younger care staff might encounter from older people who feel uncertain about their ability to properly attend to and support their care needs.

Attitudes towards older people

There is a deep-rooted cultural attitude to ageing, where older people are often presented as incapable and dependent. This highlights the need for policy-makers and those who plan and deliver public services to consider the impact of ageism (CHAI 2006). Schaie (1993: 49) provides a useful definition of ageism as:

> *a form of culturally based bias that involves restrictiveness of behaviour or opportunities based on age, age-based stereotyping, and distorted perception ... a cultural belief age is a significant dimension by definition and that it defines a person's social position, psychological characteristics or individual experience ...*

This definition highlights the relevance of a person's chronological age with regards to other people's perceptions. Expectations and thoughts about what a certain age signifies will henceforth influence our subsequent reading of that person. The following quote provides a reminder of how attitudes can influence healthcare relationships: 'Specific ageist assumptions about older people are legion: they can't hear, they can't remember, they can't think for themselves, they are depressing, they are non-productive and they are infantile' (Greene *et al.* 1986: 113).

An earlier interpretation by Cummings and Henry (1961) described 'disengagement theory' by proposing that older people progressively withdraw from social interaction as a preparation for death. Since the 1980s there had been a growing awareness of how the experience of old age has been influenced by social problems and conditions. The notion of old people potentially becoming a burden within society was being considered over a decade ago and the *Social Trends* report predicting dependant populations in 2025 concluded that there would be less children and many more elderly people, so reducing the demand for education but increasing the burden on health services (HMSO 1998). The UK has an increasingly ageing population with growth not occurring evenly across the age groups. This population trend has continued and over the last decade the number of people aged 65 and over in the UK has grown by 6 per cent, from 9.2 million in 1997 to 9.8 million in 2007. Over the next ten years this older population is projected to grow by a further 23 per cent to 12.1 million by 2017 (ONS 2009: 43).

Activity 4.4

Complete the sentences below.

➡ 'My attitudes towards older people are … '
➡ 'These values suggest … '

The *Living Well into Later Life* report identified that there is a deep-rooted cultural attitude towards ageing, where older people are often presented as incapable and dependent, especially in the media (CHAI 2006). Television media has produced numerous comedy programmes that have explored (or exploited) ageist storylines that question the competence and tolerance of the main characters. Some are listed below.

- Private Godfrey – doddering and with a weak bladder (*Dad's Army*).
- Victor Meldrew – cantankerous and argumentative (*One Foot in the Grave*).
- Father Jack – revolting and aggressive (*Father Ted*).
- Joannie Taylor – abusive and offensive (*The Catherine Tate Show*).

These well-established stereotypical portrayals and memorable catchphrases (i.e. 'I don't believe it') entertain us while at the same time highlighting the characters' incompetence, excitability and annoying behaviours. As Marshall (1990: 31) reflects, older people in sitcoms tend to promote stereotypes who are: 'enfeebled, vague and forgetful or at the other extreme cantankerous old battle-axes'. The steady flow of portrayals such as these therefore serves to reinforce views about older people as inept, disagreeable and unable to cope when faced with difficulties.

Exercise 2: Age and ageism

This exercise encouraged healthcare students to explore issues relating to their own age and factors that could contribute to the development of ageist attitudes (full details are provided in Chapter 9). It involved completing three sentences concerning the notion of age and discussing them with other group members:

- My thoughts and feelings about the age I am ...
- What I think about people who are 30 years older ...
- What age do I consider that a person becomes 'old' ...

Groups were allocated according to the decades within which students were born (i.e. 1960s, 1970s, 1980s and 1990s). This was an insightful exercise which enabled students to consider perceptions about their own age, their values, beliefs and attitudes about older people and the point at which the term 'old' can prefix a person. Discussions were lively, with some thought-provoking reflections about the concept of age being made. General feedback is included below with, for ease of reference, participants' comments being represented in two groups according to decades of birth: 1960s and 1970s, and 1980s and 1990s.

- *My thoughts and feelings about the age I am:* 60s and 70s – content with life, many responsibilities (i.e. family, mortgage), number of achievements; 80s and 90s – lots to learn, like partying, very active.
- *What I think about people who are 30 years older:* 60s and 70s – starting to slow down, things still to offer; 80s and 90s – old, 'past it'.
- *What age do I consider that a person becomes 'old':* 60s and 70s – range between 55 and 65; 80s and 90s – range between 45 and 60.

It was noted through this exercise that generational differences became evident with distinctive comments made relating to lifestyle, comfort with one's present age and feelings about getting 'old'. It appeared that younger participants viewed old people as less productive, something that was quickly countered by older participants citing notable role models such as Nelson Mandella and Clint Eastwood. This led to an interesting debate whereby certain occupational spheres such as the creative arts appeared on the whole to be more accommodating of older age, a concept that becomes equated with the notion of *experience*.

In 2005, Age Concern published *How Ageist is Britain?*' after canvassing the views and opinions of 1,843 people. One of the questions was 'What is the meaning of old?' (when do people think old age starts and youth ends). See Box 4.1 for details.

Box 4.1 How ageist is Britain?

When do people think old age starts and youth ends?

Age group	Age at which old age starts	Age at which youth ends
16–24	54.8	37.6
25–34	54.8	45.1
35–44	62.0	49.9
45–54	65.4	51.0
55–64	66.7	53.8
65–74	67.7	56.3
75+	72.0	58.0

(Age Concern 2005)

From the table provided, do you notice any patterns emerging when comparing each of the age groups?

Healthcare attitudes and older people

The *National Service Framework for Older People* (DoH 2001) identified certain concerns which professionals need to address when providing care to older people. It acknowledged the extent to which care provision has shifted away from philosophies of care that promote patient independence and lessen discrimination. Although people aged 65 and over make up only 16 per cent of the population, they occupy almost two thirds of general and acute hospital beds and account for 50 per cent of the recent growth in emergency admissions (CHAI 2006). The key findings from *Living Well into Later Life* were disconcerting as they highlighted that in spite of a number of implemented changes ageism remains across all services. This is evidenced by:

- patronizing and thoughtless treatment from staff;
- the failure of some mainstream public services, such as transport, to take the needs and aspirations of older people seriously;
- poor standards of care on general hospital wards, including poorly managed discharges from hospitals, being repeatedly moved from one ward to another for non-clinical reasons, being cared for in mixed-sex bays or wards and having meals taken away before they had been eaten due to a lack of support at meal times;
- the organizational division between mental health services for adults of working age and older people resulting in the range of services available differing for each of these groups – older people who have made the transition between these services when they reach 65 have said that there were noticeable differences in the quality and range of services available.

This interim report was based around concerns initially highlighted by the *National Service Framework for Older People*. These concerns were diverse, demeaning and arguably demoralizing as the new millennium identified strategies for:

- rooting out age discrimination;
- providing person-centred care;
- promoting older people's health and independence;
- fitting services around people's needs.

Activity 4.5

➡ What types of attitudes and behaviours shown towards older people could have encouraged the above concerns?

Attitudes and the person with dementia

Sabat and Harré (1992) described the social construction of dementia, arguing that a sense of self is still retained by the person but the public self can be lost if others fail to acknowledge it. They concluded that the attitudes and behaviours shown by other people can negate the person's sense of self if they ignore or demean it. Common discriminatory views about people with dementia see them as helpless, incapable and uncommunicative. The resultant treatment or care provided may be disempowering, ignoring a person's remaining capabilities and ability to express their needs. If the person with dementia no longer has a 'voice' with which to express themselves they can feel marginalized in the decision-making process and social conventions of dignity and respect can become undermined. In such situations a self-fulfilling prophecy can develop where the person perceives their responses to be futile and adopts more of a docile or passive stance. Withdrawing from expressing feelings about their felt experience can help to foster a cycle of dependency and enhanced feelings of disempowerment.

The conclusions of a study providing culturally sensitive services identified that professionals arranging packages of care for older eastern European people with dementia and their family carers need to become aware of the impact that earlier trauma has on them: 'Each of the carers and people with dementia were deeply affected by war experiences ... keeping it in the family ... was a symbol of survival' (Mackenzie 2006: 239). The stigma of dementia was perceived in South Asian family carer groups as tending to be linked to religious beliefs. As a result, dementia could bring about fear and jeopardize family honour and reputation, being understood as a punishment from God or that symptoms of dementia were evidence of a powerful curse (Mackenzie 2006). This all highlights the need to understand more about the person who presents with dementia and to comprehend what their past experiences and cultural views are. The more that is known about the person the more we are able to place observed behaviours or current expressions within their proper context. This means challenging stereotypical notions such as 'people with dementia can't express themselves' where any unwanted or misunderstood behaviour is regarded merely as a symptom or product of their dementia.

Case Study 4.1 reintroduces you to Elsie and considers attitudinal beliefs engendered through visiting her in her own environment. It should be noted that the following information relates to the observations made by a healthcare student and is taken from a point in time when she was still living at home, shortly before her admission into residential care.

Case Study 4.1 Elsie

To recap: Elsie is an 83-year-old woman with dementia. She had previously been an outgoing person, occupied with many activities and with a passion for animals (she worked as a veterinarian and kept a range of pets). She has fluctuating periods of lucidity and has on occasion been incontinent. She mobilizes with difficulty.

Elsie

I was asked to visit Elsie at home as she was beginning to experience early signs of Alzheimer's disease. Often reluctant to engage with health and social care services she is currently being supported in the community by a community psychiatric nurse (CPN). The CPN is well aware of her present health situation and living conditions.

Elsie lives in her own home and this was the second occasion I had visited her. On entering her home I was adamant that I was not going to sit on the furniture and would decline a drink if offered. The living room had an unpleasant smell (urine and decaying food), with signs of dirtiness (old papers strewn over the room and piles of dirty washing). I felt uncomfortable on greeting Elsie.

A visitor entering Elsie's home may feel apprehensive and uneasy when noticing the negative state of the environment. Subsequent opinions and possible concerns about her lifestyle and overall sense of well-being can be strongly influenced by this. You may find it difficult to form an appraisal about Elsie's ability to cope because of the limited amount of information provided, but certain judgements about her capability can be made (see Activity 4.6).

Activity 4.6

➡ What are your initial thoughts about Elsie and her lifestyle?
➡ If you were the carer in the above scenario, would you have similar or different attitudes and behaviours on entering her home?

We need to first understand how Elsie is coping at home even though the signs may point towards a state of not coping. What we don't know at this stage is what is usual or 'normal' for Elsie and the extent to which living circumstances have now changed following the onset of dementia. Although her lifestyle choices and lack of diligence in maintaining a tidy and habitable house may differ from your personal standards this does not necessarily mean that she is unable to care for herself. While a measure of support can be offered – i.e. with laundry and provision of meals – it needn't be assumed that she is no longer able to cope independently. However, there are potential problems with regard to how other people (i.e. neighbours) might react to a deteriorating state of cleanliness. As Smith (2001) outlines, squalor is often repellent, can represent a public health hazard and can lead to poor or antagonistic relationships with neighbours, as well as conflict with a host of agencies. This poses a dilemma and can have serious repercussions in trying to satisfy ethical tensions and professional concerns. It means finding an appropriate balance between maintaining Elsie's autonomy and self-determination rights and imposing social (including legislative) controls to safeguard her, her neighbours and the neighbourhood. Professional factors relevant to Elsie's lifestyle will be further explored in Chapter 8. Practice recommendations concerning the student's responses to Elsie are provided in Best Fit 4.1.

Best Fit 4.1

Healthcare students' responses to Elsie

- Encourage discussion on how she is coping with daily activities.
- Advise her about the general condition of her house and possible health implications.
- Appropriately challenge the way she is choosing to live in this environment.
- Offer to liaise, if Elsie agrees, with other services.
- Maintain a non-judgemental approach, using language and interpersonal behaviour that does not infer personal opinions.

Healthcare students' response to the CPN

- Report (document/verbal) what was discussed and the advice offered to Elsie.
- Describe what was observed (objectively) with regard to the condition of the living environment.
- Discuss personal values and opinions and how this has impacted upon developing a relationship with Elsie.

Observations such as those addressed above with Elsie can significantly influence the health professional's judgement of how a person with dementia views their present situation and how they live their life. Professional judgements can potentially challenge personal values and Johnson and Webb (1995: 474), as part of their conclusions on 'rediscovering unpopular patients', 'believe that social judgement has a part to play in the way we make moral decisions. We judge the social worth of individuals when balancing competing claims on our time and for our health resources'. Allied to these initial sensory evaluations a person's observed behaviours can strongly impact upon professional judgement including the extent to which we feel that the person is able to attend to their own care needs. This could ultimately influence how the person with dementia's self-determination rights are viewed and whether professional involvement becomes imposed. Healthcare interventions may necessitate listening to, supporting and encouraging, advising and instructing, challenging and educating and in certain circumstances assisting the patient with their personal care. We might use a variety of physical, psychological and social approaches to help meet this person's needs and our actions are hopefully borne out of genuine and supportive attitudes. Sometimes however we may have developed pre-judgements about the person with dementia along with their lifestyle and their behaviours. In these circumstances the attitudes we hold can be pejorative as we are focused more on a person's inabilities and deficits than what they are actually able to do.

Making judgements

The more that is known about a person's past experiences and lifestyle choices the better we are able to appreciate the whole person. At a fundamental level this can help to determine the initial phase of understanding and establishing a relationship based upon the ways the person has lived their life. What we might periodically find is that we are influenced in our judgements about others by virtue of the facts we learn about them and how they choose to live their lives. The initial appraisal of another's situation can evoke a range of emotions and in some cases engender feelings of sympathy and a need to be more nurturing and caring while in others we may feel less compassionate and more judgemental. Activity 4.7 presents two separate individuals and asks you to consider the resultant attitudinal response which may be fostered by the information provided.

Activity 4.7

Bill is in his mid-seventies and has experienced a lifetime of enduring and severe mental health problems of a depressive nature, including delusional ideas that encourage him to disengage from professional assistance. He is socially isolated from other people, chooses to live alone and is preoccupied with persecutory thoughts (people wishing to do him harm). Recently Bill has been diagnosed with dementia.

Sheila is in her early fifties and has always been socially active with a number of friends who she meets regularly in local clubs and restaurants. Weekdays often involve social drinking with work colleagues and more sustained alcohol consumption (including binge drinking) at weekends. This lifestyle has progressed throughout her adult life, each week drinking far in excess of the recommended units of alcohol. Recently she has started to become forgetful, experiencing physical disturbances, and is increasingly hostile, unco-operative and suspicious towards advice from health professionals. Sheila has been diagnosed with an early form of dementia.

➡ What are your initial impressions about Bill's present health status?
➡ What are your initial impressions about Sheila's present health status?

You might in your responses to Activity 4.7 have considered certain precipitating factors when contemplating Bill and Sheila's current state of health, including additional health problems or lifestyle choices. Bill, we learn, was already living with a considerable burden of mental health problems before his 'load' was increased with the addition of dementia. Sheila on the other hand has her alcoholic over-indulgence as a potential factor in her recent diagnosis of dementia. The attitudes and values we formulate towards other people can be influenced by the ways in which we view their past and present lifestyles, the types of judgement we make about their emotional and physical vulnerabilities and the ways in which that person views their world. Depression and dementia are often seen as co-morbid conditions that have similar presentations, with nearly a third of patients referred for dementia actually suffering from depression (Maynard 2003). This highlights the need for effective assessment in order to separate out the various components which may otherwise confuse the diagnostic process. It might be that Bill's advancing age has led in part to his presenting features to be considered as a form of dementia. Our feelings about Bill are more inclined to be sympathetic, with his being regarded as an unfortunate victim of a string of mental health problems. Sheila on the other hand could be regarded differently as we learn that she has, through her own volition, placed her body under considerable strain through her chosen lifestyle and her dementia may in some part be related to her alcohol consumption. Gupta and Warner (2008) indicate that given the neurotoxic effects of alcohol and the inexorable increase in per capita consumption, future generations may see a disproportionate increase in alcohol-related dementia. A rhetorical question you may ask yourself therefore is the amount of responsibility held by either party in relation to their present health conditions.

Reframing behaviour

The media remains a powerful resource for transmitting stereotypes and this is evident in its coverage of Alzheimer's disease and dementia. As Kirkman (2006) illustrates, people living with Alzheimer's disease are represented as victims of the disease as well as victims of the health service. One of the most noticeable aspects here relates to the particular phrasing used when referring to individuals and their behaviour. The language used in relationship-building can also reflect the status differentials that may exist: 'condescending forms of language towards the elderly, are said to be an attempt to reconcile the caring approach that nurses are expected to have, while actually operating in a controlling manner and adopting the role of parent' (Kenwright 1998: 28).

Activity 4.8 explores the use of language (sometimes pejorative and certainly stereotypical) and encourages a focus upon specific sentiments with an opportunity to reframe them in a more positive way. This activity provides opportunities to look again at initial interpretations and replace them with new thoughts and understanding.

Activity 4.8

Look at the following three statements and write down:

➡ Your initial thoughts.
➡ Your reframed thoughts (what you think might be behind the person's behaviour).

a) 'The person with dementia keeps checking the windows and doors and I can't get them to desist with this.'

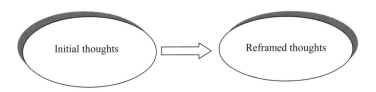

Initial thoughts → Reframed thoughts

b) 'I'm getting fed up with the aimless pacing by individuals on the ward.'

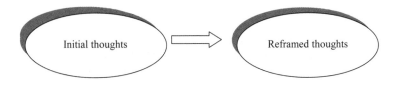

Initial thoughts → Reframed thoughts

c) 'The person with dementia started shouting at me for no reason.'

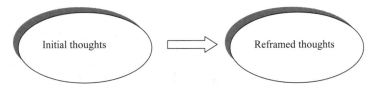

Initial thoughts → Reframed thoughts

It is interesting to look at how our view of the other person changes along with our renewed sense of comprehension about what they might be feeling or experiencing. Our attitudes can undergo a significant shift from feeling irritated or frustrated by the behaviour of the other person to feeling real compassion and understanding. What is acknowledged here is that there actually is a reason behind *all* behaviour, the problem being that we do not at the time know what it is. Potential reframing regarding the statements in Activity 4.8 could include:

a) 'The person with dementia keeps checking the windows and doors and I can't get them to desist with this.'

- It provides a sense of security.
- It relates to an activity they used to do as part of their employment.
- It is a reassuring activity because it was the last duty they did each night when living in their own home.

b) 'I'm getting fed up with the aimless pacing by individuals on the ward.'

- Pacing is never aimless.
- The patients feel restless and agitated.
- Not being able to leave the ward, the patients feel stifled and constricted.

c) 'The person with dementia started shouting at me for no reason.'

- The person is in pain or discomfort.
- The person is frustrated or feels helpless.
- The person *actually does* have a reason to be angry with me.

This highlights the importance of being able to question our initial observations and consider the range of internal experiences which might be fuelling certain behaviours. It moves us away from instinctive responses which help us to cope with our own felt experience (i.e. feeling irritated, annoyed or intimidated) towards responses which are geared more to acknowledging and addressing the feelings of those with dementia (i.e. helpless, scared and in need of comfort).

Conclusion

This chapter has explored the way in which attitudes are constructed and held about various groups in society. It has been particularly focused upon the process of double discrimination which relates to the negative set of beliefs and values commonly directed towards those who are elderly or experiencing dementia. To some degree, attitudes are created through the type of experiences we encounter when engaged in dementia care and can be mixed, with both positive and negative attributes. This is in part governed by the type of environment in which we deliver care, the qualities of the healthcare staff we work alongside and the prevailing culture of care. It can also be influenced by the individuals we are providing care for and the particular nature of their health needs. Recognizing how discriminatory attitudes develop is important and we can consider the many cases where they may be based upon erroneous assumptions or incomplete understanding. A number of ways of challenging these has been explored within this chapter including the reframing of initial interpretations, questioning concerns about care and learning more about those we are caring for.

Key points

- The attitudes we hold about others are influenced by both internal and external factors.
- We need to be mindful about our attitudes and feelings towards those who are elderly and ways in which these might impact upon care.
- It is important to recognize how we care for people with dementia based upon our feelings and expectations relating to this condition.
- The appraisal of a person's health needs and difficulties needs to be balanced against an awareness of their remaining abilities and capacity for new learning.
- In order to better appreciate and understand people with dementia we need to be cognizant of their past lifestyles and the way in which they interpret their present world.
- Opportunities for the person with dementia to express their attitudes and feelings should be facilitated so that their self-concept is not 'lost' or 'minimized'.

References

Age Concern (2005) *How Ageist is Britain?* England: Age Concern Research Services.

Alzheimer's Society (2007) *Dementia UK: The Full Report.* London: Alzheimer's Society.

Bandura, A. (1973) *Aggression: A Social Learning Analysis.* Englewood Cliffs, NJ: Prentice-Hall.

Bond, J. (1992) The politics of caregiving: the professionalization of informal care, *Ageing and Society*, 12: 5–21.

Brew, B. (2001) *HIV Neurology.* New York: Oxford University Press.

Butler, R. (1969) Ageism: another form of bigotry, *The Gerontologist*, 9: 243.

Butler, R. (1987) Ageism, in *The Encyclopaedia of Ageing.* New York: Springer.

CHAI (Commission for Healthcare Audit and Inspection) (2006) *Living Well into Later Life: A Review of Progress Against the National Service Framework.* London: DoH.

Cohen, M. (1982) *Charles Horton Cooley and the Social Self in American Thought.* New York: Garland.

Crocker, J., Major, B. and Steele, C. (1998) Social stigma, in D. Gilbert, S. Fiske and G. Lindzey (eds) *The Handbook of Social Psychology*, 4th edn. New York: McGraw-Hill.

Cummings, E. and Henry, W. (1961) *Growing Old.* New York: Basic Books.

DoH (Department of Health) (2001) *National Service Framework for Older People*. London: HMSO.

Fishbein, M. and Ajzen, I. (1975) *Belief, Attitude, Intention and Behaviour: An Introduction to Theory and Research*. Reading, MA: Addison-Wesley.

Goffman, E. (1963) *Stigma: Notes on the Management on Spoiled Identity*. London: Prentice-Hall.

Greene, M.G., Adelman, R., Charon, S. and Hoffman, S. (1986) Ageism in the medical encounter: an exploratory study of the doctor–elderly patient relationship, *Language and Communication*, 6: 113–24.

Gupta, S. and Warner, J. (2008) Alcohol-related dementia: a 21st century silent epidemic, *British Journal of Psychiatry*, 192: 351–3.

HMSO (1998) *Social Trends*. London: HMSO.

Johnson, M. and Webb, C. (1995) Rediscovering the unpopular patient: the concept of social judgement, *Journal of Advanced Nursing*, 21: 466–75.

Kenwright, T. (1998) Terms of endearment, *Kai Tiaki: Nursing New Zealand*, December/January: 28–9.

Kirkman, A. (2006) Dementia in the news: the media coverage of Alzheimer's disease, *Australian Journal of Ageing*, 25(2): 74–9.

Lippman, W. (1922) *Public Opinion*. New York: Harcourt, Brace.

Link, B. and Phelan, J. (2001) Conceptualizing stigma, *Annual Review of Sociology*, 27: 363–85.

Mackenzie, J. (2006) Stigma and dementia: East European and South Asian family carers negotiating stigma in the UK, *Dementia*, 5: 233–47.

Marshall, M. (1990) Attitudes to age and ageing, in E. McEwen (ed.) *Age: The Unrecognised Discrimination*. London: Age Concern.

Maynard, C. (2003) Differentiate depression from dementia, *The Nurse Practitioner*, 28(3): 18–27.

ONS (Office for National Statistics) (2009) *Population Trends*, No. 136. Newport: ONS.

Oskamp, S. (1977) *Attitudes and Opinions*. Englewood Cliffs, NJ: Prentice-Hall.

Rosenberg, M.J. and Hovland, C.I. (1960) *Attitude Organization and Change: An Analysis of Consistency among Attitude Components*. New Haven, CT: Yale University Press.

Sabat, S. and Harré, R. (1992) The construction and deconstruction of self in Alzheimer's disease, *Ageing and Society*, 12: 443–61.

Schaie, K. (1993) Ageist language in psychological research, *American Psychologist*, 48: 49–51.

Smith, S. (2001) Shit is good: mental health social work with lives of squalor, *Journal of Social Work Practice*, 15(1): 37–56.

Turk, V., Dodd, K. and Christmas, M. (2001) *Down's Syndrome and Dementia: Briefing for Commissioners*. London: The Mental Health Foundation.

5 The environment of care

Objectives: After reading this chapter you should be able to:

➡ Discuss how a person's environment can influence their overall sense of well-being.
➡ Explore how care approaches differ between the person's own home and the healthcare setting.
➡ Reflect upon ways to adapt or maintain a person's living space to make it conducive to well-being.

Clinical problems (the practitioner's perspective)

'I find I relate differently to people in their own homes than in the healthcare setting.'

'We are struggling to look after residents' personal items and so have to lock some of them away for safe keeping.'

'I know we could have more activities here but we don't really have the time, staff or resources.'

And yet ... attending to the person's environment can have a significant effect upon their overall sense of well-being and reduce some of the observed symptoms of dementia.

Introduction

This chapter considers the types of environment within which people with dementia live and the extent to which these environments impact upon their sense of well-being or ability to cope. The importance of a person's social setting should not be underestimated and the right kind of environment can play a major role in sustaining a person's abilities and level of independence (Cox 1998). We can start by considering the variety of settings where dementia care takes place, which include hospitals, clinics, residential homes, daycare services and the person's own home. To simplify this and for the purposes of comparison the distinction between care settings in this chapter will be between:

- a person's own home; and
- a residential healthcare setting.

Activity 5.1

➡ What do you feel are the differences between caring for a person with dementia in *our* place (healthcare setting) or *theirs* (own home)?

When healthcare occurs in a person's own home the professional worker, even though engaging in similar assessment and treatment interventions, retains a *visitor* status, having been invited into that environment. This grants a measure of control to those residing in the property and encourages a greater awareness of the need for permission-seeking on the part of the healthcare practitioner. When we call at the person's home, for example, we wait to be asked in and follow this by negotiating any interventions subsequently offered. In residential settings, however, there may be occasions when practitioners are less mindful, such as entering a person's bedroom without knocking or engaging residents in interventions without appropriate consultation – for example, by saying 'Come on Fred, you need to go to the toilet,' at the same time as helping the patient to his feet. As illustrated in Figure 5.1, the balance of power is tilted more favourably towards those who might claim ownership of the environment where care is offered. It is significantly influenced by:

- the sense of familiarity one has within an environment;
- the degree of control over aspects such as layout, routines and people chosen to share one's living space with.

First impressions

It is interesting to consider the impression that is made upon healthcare professionals and those experiencing dementia when first entering the other's environment. The person's home provides the healthcare professional with a vast storehouse of biographical information concerning lifestyle, interests, health demeanor and abilities. The healthcare professional entering a person's home will form an impression of their ability to cope. A homely, tidy and comfortable setting will create a vastly different impression to one that is cluttered, dirty and chaotic. However, not really knowing a person's usual behaviour makes it difficult to correctly contextualize our observations. While a kitchen full of dirty plates and out of date food might raise concerns about a person's cognitive ability, the same environmental observations might be made for example in some shared student residences. On the other hand, we must not ignore the impression formed by the person with dementia on entering a healthcare environment and their subsequent feelings or anxieties about care.

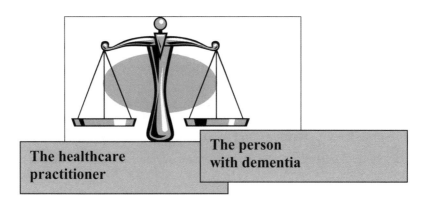

Influenced by:

- Ownership
- Familiarity
- Choice
- Control
- Resources

Figure 5.1   The balance of power

Activity 5.2

Choose an environment where you have worked with individuals experiencing dementia and consider your first impressions with regards to:

➡ Sights
➡ Sounds
➡ Smells

What were your overall feelings about the environment visited?

Activity 5.2 relates to the sensations experienced when first entering environments within which people with dementia reside. Whether or not this impression was favourable, you have no doubt been left with a related feeling about those involved and their capacity to cope. When offering this activity to healthcare students there were some starkly contrasting responses. Favourable responses included:

- *sights* – purposeful activity, personalized space, objects, pictures, brightness;
- *sounds* – conversations, music, peace and quiet;
- *smells* – flowers, fresh air, essential oils.

Unfavourable responses included:

- *sights* – clutter, mess, old food, sparseness, inactivity;
- *sounds* – wailing, shouting, overloud television/radio, telephones ringing;
- *smells* – urine/faeces, overpowering air freshener, staleness.

Activity 5.3

If you lived within an environment that exuded favourable stimuli how might you:

➡ Feel about yourself?
➡ Behave towards others?
➡ Interact with the environment?

If you lived within an environment that had unfavourable stimuli how might you:

➡ Feel about yourself?
➡ Behave towards others?
➡ Interact with the environment?

The social environment

The environment of care has a number of constituent factors which encompass much more than simply physical characteristics. We might for example consider the combined aspects of:

- the physical environment (resources, décor, layout);
- people (carers, other residents, healthcare staff or absence of people);
- the environmental culture (routines and practices).

The diversity here reflects more of a holistic feel, as reflected in established environmental models such as Maslow's hierarchy (1970) (see Activity 5.4).

Activity 5.4

➡ Maslow's hierarchy acknowledges a number of needs which include: a) physiological; b) safety (security); c) love and belonging; d) self-esteem; e) self-actualization. How do these needs relate to the person with dementia?

With reference to Activity 5.4 you may have found it easier to identify needs which sit at the lower levels of Maslow's hierarchy such as physiological and safety needs. As Bruce (2000) points out, in dementia care there is a tendency to put considerable time, energy and expertise into the physical aspects of care, while leaving other aspects vague and poorly defined. This might be due to the generally low expectations held regarding those with dementia or where physical needs take up a substantial amount of carers' time and energy. Despite having strong policy statements about higher level needs in many care settings there are few clear practice guidelines to ensure that they are achieved or ways to monitor what has been done (Bruce 2000). Needs such as self-actualization may appear less important when applied to those who are infirm or elderly with traditional notions of those who are able to *self-actualize* being in the prime of their life. It is however a hugely important and significant need which may be tied in with life review work or relate to specific goals within the person's capacity that can be aimed towards. In some cases, as will be covered later, these goals can be very substantial, such as writing books, campaigning or speaking at conferences.

The varied needs illustrated by Maslow can also be related to Kitwood's (1997) five overlapping elements of comfort, attachment, inclusion, occupation and identity, all of which come together in the central need for love (see Figure 5.2). It is through a person's experience of dementia and responses from others that these aspects start to become negatively affected. One point of note is that they are all interrelated and issues affecting any one of these needs will subsequently have an impact upon the others. This framework will be used to focus upon the person's experience of their environment and the subsequent influence upon their ability to cope.

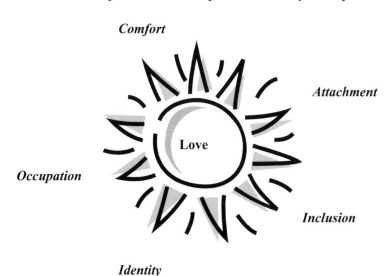

Figure 5.2 Psychological needs

Comfort

The term 'comfort' carries a number of associations encompassing physical, emotional and psychological aspects. The first-impressions activity earlier in this chapter was perhaps more attuned to physical characteristics and we might consider here the very contrasting types of setting that people reside within. A comfortable setting perhaps is bright and airy, tastefully decorated, contains appealing pictures and objects, has an abundance of plants and flowers and includes relaxing seating areas. This is very different to what is commonly found in some residential care facilities which might be characterized by a stark and sterile living space, linoleum floors, plastic-covered chairs and an absence of pictures, plants and personalized objects. All of these contribute significantly to a person's overall concept of well-being.

Activity 5.5

➡ What does *well-being* mean to you?
➡ How do you attend to your own well-being needs regarding what you do:
➡ By yourself?
➡ With other people?
➡ To your environment?

Activity 5.5 asked you to consider firstly what the term well-being means to you and secondly ways in which you maintain it. You might have considered aspects such as feeling physically and psychologically fit and healthy, being safe and secure, having supportive friends and family close by, attaining goals, being financially stable or generally feeling relaxed. A core issue relating to how we attend to our well-being needs concerns the degree of freedom or control that we have to act upon them. If feeling tense and stressed, for example, we might run a warm bath, have a glass of wine or go out for a walk. When feeling upset we have avenues open to us including seeking out supportive friends or family members for reassurance. What is key here is the range of options open to us and the say we have in acting upon them.

Activity 5.6

Think about occasions where you are in an unfamiliar environment and:

➡ are restricted from having the freedom to attend to your well-being needs;
➡ unable to influence or determine your needs.

How does this make you feel?

The feelings when not able to facilitate one's own well-being needs can cover a plethora of emotions from mild irritation to extreme distress. A long train or plane journey, for example, greatly restricts our movement and can make us increasingly restless and impatient. We might also struggle when not in our own home and wanting to retreat away from excessive noise and activity but having nowhere quiet to go. These problems are exacerbated when personal control is restricted, something commonly experienced by those with dementia. In this case, lowered expectations, fears of risk, declining abilities, isolation and environmental constraints pose significant obstacles.

The issues relating to comfort will now be addressed by looking at the *marks of well-being* as identified by Kitwood and Bredin (1992).

Exercise 1: Marks of well-being

Healthcare students were given the *marks of well-being* factors and asked to group them in priority of importance (full details of these and this exercise are provided in Chapter 9). Three categories were given which were:

- absolutely essential;
- very important;
- less important.

The choice of wording for the categories assigned a measure of importance for each of them. Justification was then sought as to why certain categories were chosen. It was interesting to note some of the issues cited over the placing of these statements including the person's level of cognitive ability (whether mild or severe dementia) or contextual environmental considerations. For example, *helpfulness* was initially considered to be less important for frail elderly individuals in moderate to severe stages of dementia, although later contended with the view that it might be a vital element for the person concerned in order to maintain a sense of purpose and feeling of value. The most commonly cited items as *absolutely essential* were those involving self-expression of needs and emotions, which were regarded as vital for all areas of care.

When trying to assign values to some of the well-being statements it is worth considering potential differences of opinion that might exist where our own frame of reference is placed over that of others (see Figure 5.3) and we have no firm guarantee that the other person's wishes are being represented. What we feel to be vital to our own well-being may differ significantly from what is felt to be important by others. For example, when feeling restless or agitated one person busies himself with strenuous physical activity while someone else chooses to listen quietly to music. We should therefore not assume that our choices or thoughts necessarily match those of the individuals we are trying to help. Recommendations for practice are provided in Best Fit 5.1.

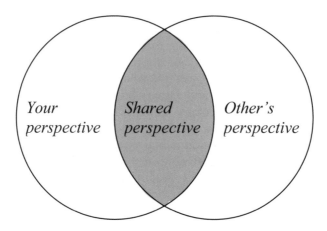

Figure 5.3 Frames of reference

Best Fit 5.1

- Don't make 'assumptions' about others' needs – take time to facilitate expression and offer choices.
- Provide opportunities for independently fulfilling needs – i.e. getting self a drink.
- Attend to the aesthetics of the environment and make it as homely as possible.

Attachment

Attachment is a fundamental requirement, a need shared by people of all ages and health states. According to Bowlby (1998) we are essentially social beings with a powerful need to maintain personal security through feeling connected to others. Indeed, the relationships a person has can be acknowledged as potentially the most important feature in maintaining their well-being (Robinson and Banks 2005). We normally have our own strategies and methods which help us to feel connected with others although can experience occasions when these are blocked or restricted. It might be, for example, that those we seek to confide in are temporarily unavailable; we are ill and unable to go out socializing; or we are experiencing technical problems and unable to phone or email friends or family. Any of these issues can cause extreme frustration and discomfort although can be accommodated if the disruption is temporary. What causes major impact is when the problem becomes prolonged, for example through illness or the death of a close friend or family member.

The difficulties facing the person with dementia are normally of a progressive nature with multiple losses of ability, decreasing social contact and lowered confidence serving to enhance the perception of a shrinking world. This all reinforces feelings of isolation and insecurity with not surprisingly a need for intimacy and closeness being heightened. The need for attachment is not lessened when individuals age or become infirm and indeed it may be the case that many older people have been deprived of physical contact such as hugs and kisses over an extended period of time, increasing their sense of isolation. Kitwood and Bredin (1992) assert therefore that carers should be generous with offering contact by holding the person's hand, walking arm in arm with them, offering a kiss or providing a gentle shoulder massage. Care is required here though as some individuals may not be used to bodily contact or might fear or misconstrue it.

Doll therapy

A fairly recent innovation and one that has courted conflicting opinions is the use of 'doll therapy'. While some researchers claim that the provision of dolls and teddy bears can help those with Alzheimer's to interact with others, it is also criticized as being infantilizing (Boas 1998). This criticism reflects one of Kitwood's (1997) *malignant social psychology* factors of treating individuals patronizingly or as if they were young children. It is a view that is countered by Kessler (2007) with the feeling that residents she observed were not *playing* with dolls but actually *caring* for them. Some of the advantages were noted in a small pilot study by MacKenzie *et al.* (2006) with residents being subsequently more active, less agitated and showing greater levels of interaction with others. What is clearly important therefore for an approach such as this is its intention and the response by those concerned. While there are dangers of infantilizing people with dementia there is also a potential for stimulating the attachment need and providing feelings of comfort and security.

Activity 5.7

➡ What do you think about the use of doll therapy?
➡ What might the advantages and disadvantages be of implementing this type of therapy?

Isolation

A common problem for those with dementia and their family carers is feeling isolated as family and friends start to withdraw, uncertain as to how to respond or relate to the person's behaviour. It is similar perhaps to the distance that those recently bereaved feel from acquaintances who want to offer support yet feel uncomfortable and unsure what to say. A further problem (as addressed in Chapter 3) relates to the issue of those with dementia entering residential care and being separated from former carers and family members, a large number of whom are keen to be involved but feel sidelined with their input being discouraged by healthcare staff. Fossey (2008) looked at the need within dementia care environments to promote positive interpersonal relationships by encouraging family involvement in care home life.

When looking at feelings of attachment we should not underestimate the role played here by other people who are experiencing dementia. This is signified by Larry Rose (1996) who speaks of his great relief at meeting and corresponding with fellow Alzheimer's sufferers and the important sense he gained of not feeling alone. This sense of connection is reflected by Yalom's (1995) process of *universality*, a dynamic identified within group therapy whereby members feel that their experience and problems are shared and understood by others.

Sexual needs

A significant aspect relating to the process of attachment is that of intimacy, a concept involving physical and emotional proximity to another person – i.e. being hugged, holding hands, or sharing a conversation or activity. An aspect which remains insufficiently addressed in older adult or dementia care is that of a person's sexual needs (Archibald 2003). These basic human needs cause many healthcarers to feel embarrassment or discomfort with assumptions that they don't (or shouldn't) apply to those who are elderly or experiencing dementia. As Harris and Wier (1998: 206) assert, it is important that we as carers remain mindful of the fact that: 'Regardless of our reluctance to notice it many older adults are sexually active and onset of cognitive dysfunction does not diminish the need for intimacy, love and affection'. This sentiment is echoed by Diana Friel-McGowin (1993: 85) who writes of her need to feel loved through sexual contact: 'I desired, and physically and emotionally needed warm, passionate touch'.

Kautz *et al.* (1990) identified some of the reasons why nurses don't address sexuality needs with common myths about older people being asexual. This becomes even more notable with gay service users who tend to become part of an invisible population (Ward *et al.* 2005). Studies find most incidents of sexual expression involving male residents and female staff members (Archibald 1998; Ehrenfeld *et al.* 1999). These incidents mostly occurred during bathing and were interpreted as sexual harassment. A problem here is that our acute feelings of discomfort and displeasure at such behaviour obstruct our ability to acknowledge the subjective or emotional reality of the other person's approach. Most of us feel uneasy when considering the sexuality of those we regard as old, unattractive, disabled or dementing. Flirting, as Mace (1992) highlights, is a common behaviour which may reinforce old social roles as well as making a person feel younger and more attractive. Unfortunately, because a person's communicative ability is restricted, *clumsy* expressions or gestures might be made which are subsequently construed as inappropriate behaviour.

Archibald (1998) found that the type of behaviour observed influenced the manner of response by healthcare staff:

- *love and caring* – supportive and understanding approach by staff;
- *romantic* – staff to some extent treated those concerned like small children;

- *erotic behaviour* – staff reactions were anger, rejection and disgust (in particular relating to the protection of female residents and staff members from the male resident's advances).

Catering for these needs might involve extending freedom for sexual engagement between family members or residents, although issues such as consent need to be clearly addressed. This involves gaining an assurance that approval and permission have been granted and that vulnerable individuals are not taken advantage of. What is vital is getting to know each individual and considering their fundamental need to feel close to a fellow human being. Whether this takes a physical or an emotional form, it will help to reduce the growing sense of isolation and disconnection all too commonly felt within the condition of dementia. It is very refreshing therefore to note Tony Robinson's observation (2008: 19): '... talking to a 90-year-old woman about what she enjoyed most at her care home. She said it was when the manageress got a male stripper in last month ... it was so outrageous and at the same time brilliant ... recognising the sexuality of older people'. Recommendations for practice are provided in Best Fit 5.2.

Best Fit 5.2

- Encourage opportunities for individuals to feel close to or connected with others.
- Consider being more generous with using touch – i.e. hand-holding.
- Take time to interpret the possible feelings or needs behind sexual behaviours.

Inclusion

Involvement

As Brooker (2007) reflects, in a number of care environments people with dementia are regarded as part of the furniture, to be vacuumed around, tidied up and polished but not communicated with. We can go further to say that in many cases choices are made on their behalf and things are done to them without adequately including or involving them in their care. Inclusion and involvement of the person with dementia means offering them choice and looking for the means that will accommodate this. Assumptions are often made on the other person's part with the view that we (healthcare professionals and family carers) know best. The question as to who does indeed know best is forcefully challenged by those experiencing this condition: 'We know what needs changing; we know what works and what doesn't work. We know this because we live it 24/7, 52 weeks a year with no days off' (Branfield and Beresford 2006: 3).

Inclusion and involvement need not only relate to personal care but, as reported by Litherland (2008), can also include service development. We can learn much from the

Alzheimer's Society's (2000) National Living with Dementia programme and by considering the factors that encourage involvement. Core aspects include:

- being respected and listened to;
- a welcoming attitude;
- being given clear encouragement;
- a clear and prompt response to questions and concerns.

Choice

When giving choice it is imperative that we are mindful as to how it is offered and the response of those concerned. As Christine Bryden (2005: 103) states:

> Present information simply and clearly, with not too many choices, and encourage us to function as normal human beings. Help us to make choices in small areas of our lives so that we feel in control, and not pushed into things.

Although ...

> If you take over our lives, then it is so easy for us to withdraw into helplessness. Life is so hard anyway and you can make it so much easier for us. But in so doing ... we will lose functions daily ... Encourage us and make us feel worthwhile, still useful and valued ... We know what we want but can't say it. In my view we are not cognitively impaired but communication impaired.

What we have here therefore is:

- too much choice = feeling overwhelmed, panicky, stressed;
- too little choice = loss of function, feeling devalued.

The important thing is to get the balance right for each person. This involves *actively listening* to the person with dementia with regard to their feelings and experience of choice and not making broad assumptions. Choice gives a person a sense of control over their life and helps to maintain a level of independence. It can also be facilitated through the adoption of a collaborative way of working, as outlined by Peplau's (1988) interpersonal relations model, where decision-making is engaged in by both parties. The drastic impact of having things taken away can be linked with a profound fear of failure. As Davis (1989: 103) writes:

> I live with the imminent dread that one mistake in my daily life will mean another freedom will be taken away from me ... If a person with Alzheimer's [cooking dinner] gets caught burning something it is a severe tragedy, another marker of the progress of her incompetency for self-sufficiency.

If we are to properly enable those with dementia to express themselves then we need to ensure that a *voice* is enabled for them. As expressed earlier, awkward or poorly managed attempts are prone to being misunderstood and dismissed. As a consequence, a person's persistence with their expression becomes increasingly regarded as 'attention seeking' (see Figure 5.4).

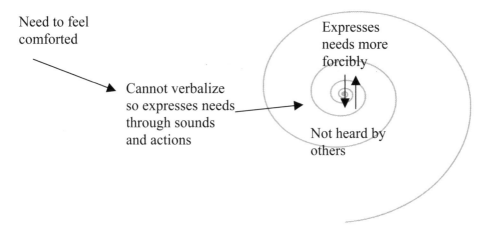

Figure 5.4   The attention-seeking spiral

Activity 5.8

Imagine yourself in the following scenarios where in each case you find it hard to adequately express your needs.

You feel hungry, having not had much to eat at breakfast as your mealtime was interrupted by your need to visit the toilet. This took longer than expected and all the breakfast items were cleared away.

It is raining and fairly cold outside yet you feel agitated and restless and wish to go for a walk. You are unable to open the door and go out.

You are in your sitting room watching and enjoying a nature programme on television. Your partner then changes the channel as it is time for Eastenders, a show you don't like.

You wish for some quiet time and personal space as you are feeling overwhelmed by all the noise and movement around you. You go to your room to lie down, yet are soon encouraged to come back to the day room as a group activity is about to commence.

➡ How do you think the person feels when unable to meet their felt needs in the above examples?

➡ What can we do to more easily discern what a person's subjective experience or immediate needs might be?

➡ What can we do to begin to address these needs and create more personal freedom for those concerned?

As Activity 5.8 shows, when prevented from meeting our periodic needs we can be left feeling frustrated and helpless. However, we are most likely unaware of the number of automatic choices we make during the course of a normal day. Our decisions are wide-ranging and cover many sub-types. For example, I might want to listen to a piece of music yet still need to determine which type, based upon my current mood: do I wish to listen to something soft and melodic or loud and rousing? The issue here is what I *feel* like doing or perhaps more significantly a contemplation of *can I be who I want to be?* Offering choice is an important aspect of person-centred care, yet within shared living environments it can pose problems whereby satisfying one person's needs impinges upon those of other people. For example, I want to listen to the radio yet others want peace and quiet; I want to go for a walk yet my partner is tired and does not want to go out. There are also environmental constraints with one interesting and perhaps debatable issue concerning the right of individuals within residential care facilities to smoke or drink.

Activity 5.9

With current laws limiting the number of premises where individuals can smoke (as well as health and safety considerations) it may be decided that residents in a care home should not be encouraged or allowed to smoke.

➡ What do you think about the introduction of such a policy?
➡ Should smoking be allowed?

Lastly, thought is needed as to how a person's spirituality or cultural needs are understood and accommodated within their environment. If wanting to pray, quiet and appropriate space is required or an opportunity to visit churches, mosques, synagogues or temples. Attention is also needed with regard to any related dietary requirements (i.e. halal or kosher) a person may have. These issues are considered in Activity 5.10. Further practice recommendations are provided in Best Fit 5.3.

Activity 5.10

Consider the following situations and what could be done to resolve them.

➡ A Muslim wishes to observe the fast during the holy month of Ramadan.

Problem: catering services are unable to provide meals after nightfall.

➡ A Jewish man wishes to celebrate Hanukkah (Festival of Lights) by the kindling of lights over eight consecutive nights.

Problem: concerns have been raised about the potential fire risk.

➡ A Sikh has had his hair washed but healthcare staff are unable to tie his turban.

Problem: there are no available relatives to help out.

➡ A Christian woman wishes to wear her crucifix.

Problem: it is an expensive item and she has inadvertently lost it on two occasions.

Best Fit 5.3

- Keep offering choices but make sure that it is done in a way which is manageable.
- Look at environmental modifications that can be made to promote freedom.
- Consider the risk behaviours a person might be restricted from alongside their potential benefits.

Occupation

It is important to recognize the influence that occupational or leisure-based activities have upon a person's well-being, such as an enhanced sense of purpose and value, engagement and connection with others, boosting one's self-esteem, feeling challenged and stimulated, having fun, feeling invigorated through exercise or peacefully relaxing. Continued involvement in activities, be they physical, cognitive or emotional, is strongly associated with healthy ageing (Bowlby 1993). A core problem for many people with dementia is the reduction or cessation of activity when reaching a level of impairment or on entering residential care. Perrin (1997) highlights the process of *occupational poverty* that exists whereby elderly people in long-term residential care are disengaged from previously valued work, leisure and self-care occupations. This also applies widely to those living at home and marks a significant shift, with inactivity being enforced upon a person through their deteriorating ability and the over-protectiveness of others. A person might be dissuaded from involvement with certain activities because of the perceived level of risk associated or even, in the case of work-based activities, because of the generalized feeling that they should 'enjoy their retirement' and 'take things easy'.

Activity 5.11

➡ How would you feel about yourself and behave towards others if you had nothing to do all day, every day?

The main issue with inactivity concerns the impact upon the person who is under-stimulated and poorly occupied. It is not a process reserved exclusively to those in residential care, and some studies highlight that a number of people living at home spend a significant amount of time unoccupied (e.g. Vikstrom *et al.* 2005). Cohen-Mansfield *et al.* (1992) demonstrate that lack of activity and occupation increase incidents of 'challenging behaviours', including wandering, agitation and aggression. What we have here is a degree of restless and pent-up energy without sufficient outlet. A vivid example of the need that individuals with Alzheimer's have for movement is provided by Robert Davis (1989: 109):

> *When the darkness and emptiness fill my mind, it is totally terrifying. I cannot think my way out of it. It stays there, and sometimes images stay stuck in my mind. Thoughts increasingly haunt me. The only way I can break this cycle is to move. Vigorous exercise to the point of exhaustion gets my mind out of the black hole ... I try to schedule my daily routine with productive, physically demanding activity. Following this I rest quietly, listening to my tapes and sometimes fall asleep. When I awake I am refreshed and usually more alert mentally.*

Imagine then restricting Robert's movement further and dissuading him from taking part in strenuous physical exertion ...

Case Study 5.1 Elsie

To recap: Elsie is an 83-year-old widower living in residential care. Before her admission she kept mentally active by doing word puzzles and crosswords but she struggles with them now due to confused thinking and poor concentration. She has fluctuating periods of lucidity and confusion, becoming extremely distressed when more aware of her deteriorating cognition.

Elsie

Reports from relatives inform us that Elsie always had a passion for puzzles, crosswords and word-search activities. These have been offered to her on a number of occasions and she appears readily enthusiastic. The problem is that after a few minutes she does not want to continue with them and appears irritated, angry and upset.

- What do you think might be Elsie's experience of this activity?
- Should we persist in offering her this?
- What should we do to help her?

One of the core issues highlighted by Case Study 5.1 is that Elsie formerly took great pleasure in and was mentally stimulated by crosswords and word puzzles but they now remind her forcibly of her failing capacity. The frustration and distress here might centre around her inability to fill in a single word on a crossword when in the past she would have been able to complete it with little difficulty. We are faced with the polarized choices of either persisting with this type of activity or doing something different. What is important is trying to find something which Elsie finds absorbing and mentally stimulating but which, crucially, matches her current capabilities.

Activity 5.12

➡ Consider the various opportunities or resources in your workplace that are open to those with dementia for engaging in purposeful or personally significant activities.

There are many activities that can be engaged in by those with dementia, and Kitwood and Bredin (1992) list cooking, dancing, flower arranging, playing games, gardening, doing housework, listening to music, going on outings, walking and religious observance. This list can be extended indefinitely given the particular needs and wishes of those involved as well as what is practicable to facilitate. An example of good practice is illustrated by Merevale House, a Warwickshire care home for younger people with dementia which provides space for quiet and tranquil reflection as well as purposeful activity – i.e. working on an allotment or in a workshop, reading books or watching DVDs. One resident reports: 'They try to cater to each person's interests here and recognize the individual. It's like interests-based care and it heightens a person's motivation' (Alzheimer's Society 2007).

Meaningful and valued occupation should not be exclusive to younger people and needs diligently pursuing for everyone regardless of age or health status. Perrin (1997) reports on the outcome of introducing 14 different types of activity to individuals with advanced dementia, with positive effects being noticed in approximately 60 per cent of cases. Activities are clearly not restricted to those with mild to moderate function and there are certain approaches that are geared towards later-stage dementia including tactile, olfactory, acoustic and visual stimulation (Calkins 1997), examples of which might include the use of multi-sensory stimulation or massage. Activities geared towards sensory stimulation reflect one of Kitwood's (1997) enhancing personhood factors, that of *timulation*. Whatever activity is offered needs to match the abilities of the person concerned as while under-stimulation can lead to apathy, restlessness and agitation, over-stimulation can be draining and confusing. The latter is illustrated by Robert Davis (1989) who became overwhelmed by a family trip to Disney World and subsequently required days of lying down in a darkened room in order to regain his sense of equilibrium. See Best Fit 5.4 for practice recommendations.

Best Fit 5.4

- Recognize the impact upon a person when:
  - under-occupied;
  - over-occupied.
- Involvement with activities should include a degree of choice.
- Make sure that activities reflect individual needs and requirements.

Identity

The condition of dementia brings with it a fundamental shift from what might be regarded as my *former self* (before diagnosis) to the ever-changing *present self*. What a person might be experiencing can be hard to ascertain and while there are a growing number of first-person accounts by individuals in the early to moderate stages of dementia, these become scarcer and more fragmented as the condition advances. Bernlef's (1988) *Out of Mind* provides a vivid account of this fragmenting process with a narrative style that becomes more disjointed and less coherent over time, thereby reflecting the terrifying prospect of losing conscious thought and awareness of self. This is reflected in Cotrell and Hooker's (2005) study investigating fears concerning advancing dementia with worries about not being aware of what's going on and one respondent stressing, 'I want to observe and feel part of life'. A common desire expressed on the Alzheimer's Society website is that of individuals with dementia seeking out friends and family to act as the guardians of their memories. The feeling here is of being provided with a measure of comfort knowing that chosen advocates will be able to represent their *essence* to others.

The gradual disappearance of personal identity also has a major impact upon carers and family members who are faced with the contemplation of a slow grieving process. John Bayley (1999 : 84) recounts the words of a fellow carer as: 'The lady told me in her own deliberately jolly way that living with an Alzheimer victim was like being chained to a corpse ... a corpse that complains all the time'. It is fortunately not a view that he held himself, managing to retain a close relationship and a high degree of fondness for the person (Iris) still residing within the condition of dementia. When looking at the notion of identity in advancing dementia it is important to replace the idea of a person disappearing with the thought of them becoming *harder to locate*. For a start, it needs to be stressed that a number of individuals in later-stage dementia still have periods of fluctuating lucidity (Normann *et al.* 2006). Not recognizing this causes carers to dismiss or be unaware of genuine attempts at communication. There is some encouraging work by Richards and Tomandl (2006) which facilitated some meaningful communication with individuals in later-stage dementia including speech, expressive gestures, hand squeezing and joining in with singing. What can be highlighted here is our need to attend more closely to what a person is communicating and to persist in communicating with them no matter what their level of impairment might be. As stressed by Kitwood and Bredin (1992: 27): 'the best thing is to treat everything they say, however jumbled or fantastic it may seem to be, as an attempt to tell us something. Look for the message that underlies the words, or a need that is being expressed'.

Activity 5.13

➡ What makes me unique and different from others?
➡ If I was no longer in a position to represent myself, what would I most like others to know?
  ➡ Who I am?
  ➡ My wishes and needs?
  ➡ My likes and dislikes?

Activity 5.13 highlights various issues which help to make us who we are. These are so fundamental to our very being that to lose them would mean stripping us of our identity. What is crucial is to retain them as far as possible no matter what stage of debilitation we find ourselves in. Collaborative work between healthcare staff and those with dementia and their carers can engage in the process of recording and retaining key aspects of a person's life. A variety of resources such as narratives, video diaries, photo albums or internet blogs could be created when cognition is still reasonably intact. Even if the person is communicatively impaired, using a range of creative and expressive activities such as poetry, singing or art might help. An interesting example relates to the encouragement of those with Alzheimer's to express themselves through painting and telling their story in a more comprehensible language (Jenny and Oropeza 1994). It might also be useful to invite family members to come and meet with care staff in order to 'present' and share their reflections about their relative.

There are some major environmental considerations to bear in mind when considering what helps to maintain a person's identity. The person living in their own home will often have multiple cues and signifiers of personality. This is conveyed through aspects such as photographs of family and friends, ornaments, furniture, books, recorded films and television programmes, or music tapes and CDs. Each of these has the potential to act as a trigger for memory. For example, a simple vase on the mantelpiece represents a memorable holiday I had with my wife in France. Each time I catch sight of photographs on the wall of children and grandchildren it gets me thinking about them and wondering what they might be currently doing. A set of well-read Dickens books on the shelf next to my chair is occasionally dipped into as I seek to enjoy some of the characters again. The core issue here is that I am able to keep sight of who I am and what is most important to me. Within residential care however this picture is less certain and many people spend their time devoid of familiar and reinforcing cues. At worst, even family photographs are not displayed and there are no items of personal significance around – i.e. books, music or ornaments. This is inexcusable and shows real neglect of the needs of those being cared for. A notable approach which was featured in the *Tonight: Kevin Whately on Dementia* programme

(ITV1, 23 March 2009) showed 'achievements' being pinned up on bedroom doors for care staff and residents to see as a frequent reminder of something of the essence of the person with dementia.

Activity 5.14

➡ What approaches (i.e. reminiscence work, tea dances, discussion groups) or resources (i.e. photograph albums, books, films) do you think help to maintain identity in those with dementia?

In Activity 5.14 you may have considered one of many approaches such as life review, creating life-history boxes, going on outings to memorable places, discussion groups around shared themes, looking at photograph albums or listening to favourite music, all of which which fit under the umbrella term of 'reminiscence'. As well as benefiting the person with dementia these approaches are hugely valuable for professional carers as knowing more about the person's background enables a better awareness of who they are in the present (Pietrukowicz and Johnson 1991; Gibson 2004; Bruce and Schweitzer 2008). This is aptly illustrated by Lauren Kessler (2007: 95) and her work in a residential facility:

> Then it starts to make sense: the way he has to know every small detail, the way he wants every process broken down into small steps, the way he can't move until he knows what's next. This must be how he lived his occupational life. This must be how he sees the world. This must be how his brain works ... the second I make that connection my impatience disappears and I begin to admire how orderly and logical Hayes is ... It also gives me a positive way of interacting with him. I will treat him like the methodical, systematic, organized engineer he was.

It was also stressed by Schweitzer and Bruce (2008) that family carers might find that revisiting the past improves their current relationship with the person cared for. This is an important point, especially with the massive caregiver strain commonly experienced (and covered in Chapter 3). Recommendations are provided in Best Fit 5.5.

Best Fit 5.5

- Ensure that those with dementia have regular access to personally reinforcing cues.
- Provide opportunities for preparing resources and material (especially in the early stages) that can help to reaffirm identity.
- Offer space for carers to 'present' their relative to healthcare staff.
- Include identity reminders within care plans and care notes.

Enhancing the environment

Exercise 2: Dimensions and the social environment

This exercise asked healthcare students to attend to environmental design by creating a new dementia care facility (full details are provided in Chapter 9). It set out to tackle some of the commonly cited problems resulting from low staffing levels and a paucity of resources. It was acknowledged that greater personal freedom needs to be balanced against risk factors, some of which can be accommodated by environmental structural design such as enclosed gardens with free access. There also needs to be clearer and easier orientation around the facility with clear signs and pictures – i.e. highlighting where the toilet or bedroom areas are. One detrimental factor noted within many care homes has been the unwelcome and irritating distractions of television and radio sounds which play throughout the day with little choice being offered. As one student noted this might be more for the benefit of the staff (citing an example from practice of Galaxy FM being chosen over more relaxing radio stations such as Radio 3 or Radio 4). This exercise challenged students to be more mindful about the overall effects of the environment upon the person with dementia.

Technology

Current attempts to promote independent living for those with dementia and their carers are assisted through the development of a range of electronic resources and devices. It is interesting to look back on modern-day devices which are in everyday use yet a few decades back were viewed as futuristic and fantastic. Some of those featured on BBC's *Tomorrow's World* programme included:

- the breathalyser (1967);
- the ATM cash machine (1969);
- the pocket calculator (1971);
- the digital watch (1972);
- Teletext (CEEFAX) (1975);
- the personal stereo (1980);
- the compact disc and player (1981);
- the camcorder (1981);
- the barcode reader (1983);
- the clockwork radio 1993.

Activity 5.15

What kind of device or technological aid do you think might appear over the next few decades to help promote independent living for people with dementia?

The present-day range of technological devices is developing rapidly with Telecare and Telehealth facilities offering a broad range of resources which facilitate living skills for those with dementia. The type of facility available can be grouped under the following headings (Atdementia 2009):

- prompts and reminders;
- leisure;
- communication;
- safety.

Prompts and reminders

Devices which act as memory prompts and reminders by providing visual, verbal or audible cues – i.e. electronic calendars, locator devices, medication reminders/dispensers and memo minders.

Leisure

These devices help support and enable leisure activities – i.e. computer aids, easy to use television and radio, reminiscence material and games.

Communication

These devices include intercoms, pre-programmed telephones/mobiles and aids that help people with dementia to take part in conversations.

Safety

Devices which can help improve safety in the person's home – i.e. activity monitors, alarms, fall detectors, flood detectors, water temperature monitors, gas, carbon monoxide, smoke and extreme temperature detectors and 'wandering' location devices.

The use of Telecare is steadily growing with some positive results being found, for example, with the Aztec Telecare Project, a joint project between the Maudsley Hospital and Croydon Council's services for those with dementia; the Smart Technology Telecare project which was implemented in West Lothian, Scotland; and the Safe at Home project, an initiative which reduced the need for residential care and helped promote independent living (Woolham 2005). These and similar projects have been helped by the government's £80 million preventive technology grant which was available over two years from April 2006. The government's aim was to reduce residential and nursing care costs as well as the burden upon family carers, and to facilitate independent living for service users (DoH 2009). Clearly something needs to be done to address this problem, especially with predicted costs for 2025 being estimated at £17 billion per year. The Alzheimer's Society is strongly supportive of these initiatives, believing that Telecare could play a significant role in helping people with dementia (Alzheimer's Society 2009).

Implications

Activity 5.16

Briefly consider what you feel might be the funding, social or ethical implications of the above technological aids.

➡ Funding implications.
➡ Social implications.
➡ Ethical implications.

As you may have considered in Activity 5.16, some of the costs may prove prohibitive and limit what can realistically be offered. There may also be a significant issue over who pays for these aids with costs being disputed between social services, healthcare agencies and the person with dementia and their family. There may also be problems encountered through the ease or difficulty of installing devices as the person's living space might not be suited for some adaptations. The reorganization might involve having to lose personal items or change environmental aspects that have sentimental or emotional significance – for example, replacing a cooking range that has been used by the family for decades with a modern gas appliance. There are also issues to consider regarding the implications of change to others – i.e. family members and carers who share that person's living space. The use of technology also raises concerns regarding its potential misuse when employed as a means of controlling or restricting behaviour. Devices such as wristbands or mobile phones with GPS tracking facilities are being used to help 'track' movement, albeit for safety purposes, but at the same time the concept of 'electronic tagging' does raise some concerns. While the Alzheimer's Society welcomes the benefits provided by this type of technology it also cautions about a person's loss of privacy and the risk of a false sense of security (Alzheimer's Society 2009). Dr Richard Nicholson, editor of the *Bulletin of Medical Ethics* raised the potential for 'second-class care' to be offered, which while making life easier for overburdened carers does not necessarily make life safer or more pleasant for the person with Alzheimer's (BBC 2007). A note of concern was expressed by Woolham (2005) who highlighted that the use of Telecare should be as an adjunct to social care rather than a substitute, because otherwise the existing loneliness and isolation felt by many people with dementia will be compounded.

Conclusion

This chapter has considered the significance of the person's living space to their sense of well-being and ability to cope with their experience of dementia. Clearly, there are major differences between the person's own home (*their* space) and designated health care facilities (*our* space) which influence attitudes and approaches to care. Other aspects covered here considered ways in which a person's holistic needs might be facilitated by their environment. This encompasses a person's total living experience including the nature of social contact encountered or the aesthetics and comfort of their living space. The core issue to bear in mind here is that a person's environment exerts a significant influence upon their overall well-being and that a number of behavioural problems or psychological difficulties subsequently observed can be directly attributed to the social setting and *not* the condition of dementia.

Key points

- Don't make assumptions – help those with dementia to express their thoughts and feelings.
- Attend to the homeliness of the environment and the degree of freedom allowed.
- Encourage opportunities for individuals to feel close to or connected with others.
- Facilitate choice-taking and personal expression no matter how cognitively impaired a person might be.
- Consider risk behaviours a person might be restricted from alongside their potential benefits.
- Ensure that a wide range of occupational activities are available and that these are geared towards individual need and personal choices.
- Ensure that those with dementia and their carers have regular access to personally reinforcing cues.

References

Alzheimer's Society (2000) *National Living with Dementia Programme*, www.alzheimers.org.uk/site/scripts/documents_info.php?categoryID=200134&documentID=468, accessed 6 October 2009.

Alzheimer's Society (2007) *Living With Dementia*, /www.alzheimers.org.uk/site/scripts/documents.php?categoryID=200241, accessed 8 November 2008.

Alzheimer's Society (2009) *Assistive Technology*, www.alzheimers.org.uk/site/scripts/documents_info.php?categoryID=200192&documentID=109, accessed 22 March 2009.

Archibald, C. (1998) Sexuality, dementia and residential care: managers' report and response, *Health and Social Care in the Community*, 6(2): 95–101.

Archibald, C. (2003) Sexuality and dementia: the role dementia plays when sexual expression becomes a component of residential care work, *Alzheimer's Care Quarterly*, 4(2): 137–48.

Atdementia (2009) *What do we Mean by Assistive Technology?*, www.atdementia.org.uk/editorial.asp?page_id=25, accessed 15 February 2009.

BBC (2007) Charity backs dementia taggings, http://news.bbc.co.uk/1/hi/health/7159287.stm, accessed 5 March 2009.

Bayley, J. (1999) *Iris: a Memoir of Iris Murdoch*. London: Abacus.

Bernlef, J. (1988) *Out of Mind*. London: Faber & Faber.

Boas, I. (1998) Why do we have to give the name 'therapy' to companionship and activities that are, or should be, a part of normal relationships?, *Journal of Dementia Care*, 6: 13.

Bowlby, C. (1993) *Therapeutic Activities with Persons Disabled by Alzheimer's Disease and Related Disorders*. Gaithersburg, MD: Aspen.

Bowlby, J. (1998) *Attachment and Loss*. London: Pimlico.

Branfield, F. and Beresford, P. (2006) *Making User Involvement Work: Supporting Service User Networking and Knowledge*. York: Joseph Rowntree Foundation.

Brooker, D. (2007) *Person-Centred Dementia Care: Making Services Better*. London: Jessica Kingsley.

Bruce, E. (2000) Looking after well-being: a tool for evaluation, *Journal of Dementia Care*, November/December: 25–7.

Bruce, E. and Schweitzer, P. (2008) Working with life history, in M. Downs and B. Bowers (eds) *Excellence in Dementia Care: Research into Practice*. Maidenhead: Open University Press.

Calkins, M. (1997) A supportive environment for people with late-stage dementia, in C. Kovach (ed.) *Late-Stage Dementia Care: A Basic Guide*. Philadelphia, PA: Taylor & Francis.

Cohen-Mansfield, J., Werner, P. and Marx, M. (1992) Observation data on time use and behaviour problems in nursing homes, *Journal of Applied Gerontology*, 11(1): 114–17.

Cotrell, V. and Hooker, K. (2005) Possible selves of individuals with Alzheimer's disease, *Psychology and Aging*, 20(2): 285–94.

Cox, S. (1998) *Home Solutions: Housing and Support for People with Dementia*. London: Housing Associations Charitable Trust.

Davis, R. (1989) *My Journey into Alzheimer's Disease*. Bucks: Tyndale House.

DoH (Department of Health) (2009) *Preventative Technology Grant*, www.dh.gov.uk/en/Publicationsandstatistics/Publications/PublicationsPolicyAndGuidance/Browsable/DH_5464107, accessed February 2009.

Ehrenfeld, M., Bronner, G., Tabak, N., Alpert, R. and Bergman, R. (1999) Sexuality among institutionalized elderly patients with dementia, *Nursing Ethics*, 6(2): 144–49.

Fossey, J. (2008) Care homes, in M. Downs and B. Bowers (eds) *Excellence in Dementia Care: Research into Practice*. Maidenhead: Open University Press.

Friel-McGowin, D. (1993) *Living in the Labyrinth: a Personal Journey through the Maze of Alzheimer's Disease.* New York: Delacorte Press.

Gibson, F. (2004) *The Past in the Present: Using Reminiscence in Health and Social Care.* Baltimore, MD: Health Professions Press.

Harris, L. and Wier, M. (1998) Inappropriate sexual behavior in dementia: a review of the treatment literature, *Sexuality and Disability*, 16: 205–17.

Jenny, S. and Oropeza, M. (1994) *Memories in the Making.* Irvine, CA: Alzheimer's Association of Orange County.

Kautz, D., Dickey, C. and Stevens, M. (1990) Using research to identify why nurses do not meet established sexuality nursing care standards, *Journal of Nursing Quality Assurance*, 4(3): 69–78.

Kessler, L. (2007) *Dancing with Rose: Finding Life in the Land of Alzheimer's.* London: Viking.

Kitwood, T. (1997) *Dementia Reconsidered: the Person Comes First.* Buckingham: Open University Press.

Kitwood, T. and Bredin, K. (1992) *Person–Person: A Guide to the Care of Those with Failing Mental Powers.* Loughton: Gale Centre.

Litherland, R. (2008) Involving people with dementia in service development and evaluation, in M. Downs and B. Bowers (eds) *Excellence in Dementia Care: Research into Practice.* Maidenhead: Open University Press.

Mace, N. (1992) *The 36 Hour Day: A Family Guide to Caring at Home for People with Alzheimer's Disease and Other Confusional Illnesses.* London: Hodder & Stoughton.

MacKenzie, L., James, I., Morse, R., Mukaetova-Ladinska, E. and Reichelt, K. (2006) A pilot study on the use of dolls for people with dementia, *Age and Aging*, 35(4): 441–4.

Maslow, A. (1970) *Motivation and Personality.* London: Harper & Row.

Normann, H., Asplund, K., Karlsson, S., Sandman, P. and Norberg, A. (2006) People with severe dementia exhibit episodes of lucidity, *Journal of Clinical Nursing*, 15(11): 1413–17.

Peplau, H. (1988) *Interpersonal Relations in Nursing: A Conceptual Frame of Reference for Psychodynamic Nursing.* Basingstoke: Macmillan Education.

Perrin, T. (1997) Occupational need in severe dementia: a descriptive study, *Journal of Advanced Nursing*, 25: 934–41.

Pietrukowicz, M. and Johnson, M. (1991) Using life histories to individualise nursing home staff attitudes towards residents, *The Gerontologist*, 31: 105–6.

Richards, T. and Tomandl, S. (2006). *An Alzheimer's Surprise Party*, www.tomrichards.com/publications.htm, accessed 1 February 2009.

Robinson, J. and Banks, P. (2005) *Care Services Enquiry: The Business of Caring.* London: King's Fund.

Robinson, T. (2008) Imagine we had just 3 days to do it, *NMC News*, 25: 18–19.

Rose, L. (1996) *Show Me the Way to go Home.* Forest Knolls, CA: Elder Books.

Vikstrom, S., Borell, L., Stigsdotter-Neely, A. and Josephsson, S. (2005) Caregivers' self-initiated support toward their partners with dementia when performing an everyday occupation together at home, *Occupation, Participation and Health*, 25(4): 149–59.

Ward, R., Vass, A., Aggarwal, N., Garfield, C. and Cybyk, B. (2005) A kiss is still a kiss? The construction of sexuality in dementia care, *Dementia: The International Journal of Social Research and Practice*, 4(1): 49–72.

Woolham, J. (2005) *The Effectiveness of Assistive Technology in Supporting the Independence of People with Dementia: The Safe at Home Project*. London: Hawker Publications.

Yalom, I. (1995) *The Theory and Practice of Group Psychotherapy*. New York: Basic Books.

Further reading

Bryden, C. (2005) *Dancing with Dementia*. London: Jessica Kingsley.

Moos, R. and Lemke, S. (1985) Specialised living environments for older people, in J. Birren and K. Schaie (eds) *Handbook of the Psychology of Aging*. New York: Reinhold.

Schweitzer, P. and Bruce, E. (2008) *Remembering Yesterday, Caring Today – Reminiscence in Dementia Care: A Guide to Good Practice*. London: Jessica Kingsley.

6   The *person* with dementia

Objectives: After reading this chapter you should be able to:

➡ Reflect upon the factors which establish a person's uniqueness.
➡ Discuss how personal differences can influence a person's individual experience of dementia.
➡ Explore ways by which interventions can be tailored to more closely fit the person you are working with.

Clinical problems (the practitioner's perspective)

'When we hear the term *person with dementia* we more often than not think about individuals in the later stages of this condition.'

'Person-centred care tends to be based upon assumptions and stereotypical notions as opposed to actual observed evidence.'

'It is hard at times to gather information about the person with dementia and I have to draw upon experiences of working with others with related difficulties.'

'We are restricted in the use of person-centred care because of limitations of time, staff and resources.'

And yet ... embracing person-centred care could both challenge traditional paternalistic ways of caring and provide greater opportunities for promoting self-determination for the person with dementia.

Introduction

The person-centred approach has featured as part of healthcare practice for a number of years now, with strong roots within the work of humanists such as Carl Rogers (1961) and Abraham Maslow (1970). It is an approach which has over the past two decades featured more prominently within dementia care, particularly due to the work by Tom Kitwood and the Bradford Dementia Group who challenged the old order of care (traditional, institutional approaches) and advocated its replacement by a more humanistic, person-centred philosophy. This work was supported by the King's Fund's (1986) publication of *Living Well Into Old Age* which set out a code of practice highlighting the rights of people with dementia. More recently, the focus on person-centred care has been advocated by a series of policy documents which include the *Living Well with Dementia: A National Dementia Strategy* (DoH 2009), the *National Service Framework for Older People* (DoH 2001), *A New Ambition for Old Age* (DoH 2006a), *Dignity in Care* (DoH 2006b) and *Securing Better Mental Health for Older Adults* (DoH 2005). These are welcome initiatives given the current climate with the majority of health and social care services for people with dementia being unable to adapt their services to be sufficiently flexible to the needs of individual people (Daker-White *et al.* 2002).

Activity 6.1

➡ What is your understanding of the term *person-centred care*?
➡ To what degree have the above initiatives influenced your experience of care delivery?

Person-centred care

Person-centred care stresses the need to acknowledge the uniqueness and individuality of each person, appreciating their particular circumstances as well as their experience of dementia. This is clearly reflected in Kitwood's (1997: 8) concept of *personhood*, a term which he defined as: 'A standing or status that is bestowed upon one human being, by others, in the context of relationship and social being'. It is also outlined in the distinction placed between the following terms:

- person with *dementia*;
- *person* with dementia.

The stress placed upon the above words reflects the degree of importance afforded them, either with the person or condition of dementia taking prominence. In order to achieve a better balance it is important to have a clearer understanding about what the condition of dementia signifies from the point of view of felt and lived experience. This brings in Naomi Feil's (2002) approach of *validation* which recognizes the subjective reality of another person's experience. The essence of this relates to who the person is and that in order to offer individual and empathic care we need to properly acknowledge and understand the various elements that make a person unique.

The term *person with dementia* perhaps first brings to mind certain assumptions and ideas about an individual's behaviour, coping skills and cognitive abilities. This might commonly incorporate stereotypical views of the confused old person who is very dependent upon others. While this might be the case it could also relate to someone in their forties or fifties who appears lucid and focused, still working and living independently. The dementia spectrum (see Figure 6.1) covers an almost infinite array of issues and capabilities and it is important to look at each person's unique experiences.

Early phase   *Middle phase*   *Later phase*

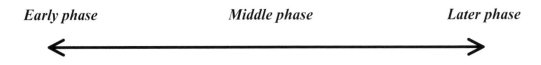

- Employed
- Drives regularly
- Lives at home
- Looks after dependants
- Active social life
- Maintains leisure interests

- Heavily dependent upon others
- Lives in residential care
- Physically frail and infirm
- Minimal contact with family and friends
- Insufficiently occupied

Figure 6.1   The dementia spectrum

'First we saw our friendly harassed GP who asked Iris who the Prime Minister was. She had no idea but said to him with a smile that it surely didn't matter' (Bayley 1999: 234). This extract is taken from John Bayley's account which observes his wife Iris's experience of dementia. It has been included here as a starting point because it succinctly sums up a crucial aspect, namely the *person* who still resides within the condition of dementia. It is something that may tend to get overlooked when a diagnosis of dementia is suspected and the subsequent barrage of cognitive assessments, brain scans and blood tests give the impression of reducing a person's multi-faceted qualities and rich individual experiences to a set of figures, images and results. All too often the person who has dementia becomes submerged not only by their present experienced symptoms and difficulties but also by the way in which they are subsequently regarded by others post-diagnosis. This is commonly deficits-based and centred around what a person is no longer able to do. We tend to speak about the person disappearing and when we are no longer able to see them the feeling is that they are no longer there. Similarities can be drawn with the small child's sensation of closing their eyes and imagining that because they can't see themselves then others can't either. Within dementia care we need to continually look for and value the *person* who still exists within the condition of dementia despite being concealed by various symptoms. This chapter addresses some of the various aspects that make people uniquely different and how these might influence their subsequent experience of dementia. This then forms the basis for considering the approach of person-centred care and its application in practice.

Activity 6.2

➡ Consider the characteristics that make *you* different from other people.

A person's uniqueness can be regarded through different dimensions such as culture, gender, temperament, social class, lifestyle, outlook, beliefs, values, commitments, tastes and interests (Kitwood 1997). In order to better understand who the person with dementia is, these aspects have been developed and included within a framework (see Figure 6.2) comprising the three separate sub-headings of:

- personal characteristics;
- associated health states;
- affiliation.

This framework is not intended as a definitive list and a number of other factors could be added. It does however start to highlight some of the multi-dimensional characteristics and features which play a part in defining who we are.

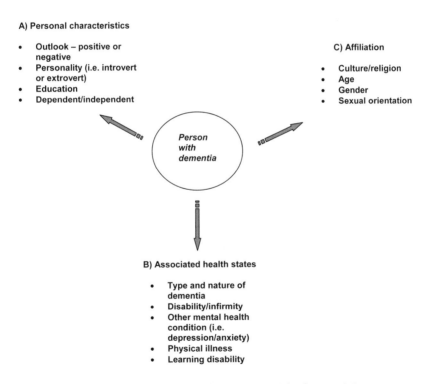

A) Personal characteristics

- Outlook – positive or negative
- Personality (i.e. introvert or extrovert)
- Education
- Dependent/independent

C) Affiliation

- Culture/religion
- Age
- Gender
- Sexual orientation

Person with dementia

B) Associated health states

- Type and nature of dementia
- Disability/infirmity
- Other mental health condition (i.e. depression/anxiety)
- Physical illness
- Learning disability

Figure 6.2 Who is the *person* with dementia?

Personal characteristics

Of interest here are the personal characteristics (i.e. personality issues or outlook on life) that help to predispose individuals towards specific responses or coping approaches, be they adaptive or maladaptive. While some people are able to maintain a degree of optimism and reframe problems as 'challenges', others become overwhelmed with feelings of pessimism, retreating away from the world or becoming increasingly dependent. There are a number of reasons why people cope in such different ways with the experience of dementia, some of which will explored in the following section and include:

- outlook (positive or negative);
- introvert or extrovert;
- education;
- dependence/independence.

Outlook (positive or negative)

The issue here concerns a person's personal framework which may predispose them either towards a positive or negative orientation. Clearly, this is not necessarily a constant factor and can change at any time in response to life events and personal issues. Recognizing what a person's outlook is need not necessarily be straightforward as there may be a tendency to label people from their behaviours – i.e. *miserable* and *grumpy* Jim or *happy* and *carefree* Agnes. These behaviours can then easily be reinforced through our subsequent dealings with Jim and Agnes as we are influenced by our expectations of them.

Within the experience of dementia, a person's outlook can come across as inspiring and encouraging. For example, Christine Bryden (2005: 170), writing about her own experience of Alzheimer's, states:

> *I choose a new identity as a survivor. I want to learn to dance with dementia. I want to live positively each day, in a vital relationship of trust with my care partners alongside me … To live with the fear of 'ceasing to be' takes enormous courage. The precious string of pearls, of memories, that is our life, is breaking, the pearls are being lost. But by finding new pearls, those created in the struggle with dementia, we can put together a new necklace of life, of hope in our future.*

These words are very expressive and positive in nature, underlining her determination to battle this condition. We can match this sense of optimism with other stories of personal achievement, examples which strongly contrast the usual stereotypes of people with dementia as helpless and dependent. The Alzheimer's Society's monthly *Living with Dementia* has many such illustrations of people post-diagnosis getting on with their life and succeeding in:

- running the London Marathon;

- writing a book;
- getting married;
- speaking at conferences.

Clearly, this does not apply to everybody and we should look at each person individually. However, it is evident that some people are able to find untapped reserves and cope with terrible afflictions, for example, the Falkland's War veteran and burns victim Simon Weston or the cancer sufferer Jane Tomlinson. The degree of optimism or pessimism felt by various individuals is dependent upon the severity of their condition, their previous outlook on life, support mechanisms and available resources. While we can regard some of the above examples as inspiring and worthy of celebration we must also recognize and respect those who don't feel inclined or motivated towards doing something amazing. It is also important to recognize the smaller events that might constitute 'amazing achievements' for the person concerned – i.e. attending a day centre, going shopping or simply expressing a desire or need.

Introvert or extrovert

An individual's personality needs to be properly appreciated in order for us to understand the significance of their mood and behaviour. One pertinent aspect concerns their location along a continuum from *introverted* to *extroverted*, as some people naturally prefer privacy and solitude while others are more in need of social engagement. An awareness of a person's predisposition is important as misinterpretations can ensue. For example, an individual might appear withdrawn and uncommunicative yet feel reasonably well and content. Without knowing much about this person we might then vigorously allocate them to various group activities in order to counter what we perceive to be their sense of isolation. This is then resisted because the person feels uncomfortable and threatened by the experience being promoted. Activity 6.3 looks at the way in which we deal with different people and addresses Moos and Lemke's (1985) study of the social environment and its impact upon those with dementia. It focuses in particular upon the need for:

- *integration* – degree to which residents are integrated into the life of the home;
- *privacy* – degree to which residents are able to separate from the community.

Activity 6.3

➡ Fill in the boxes below, considering how you might meet the needs of *integration* and *privacy* for Arthur and Elsie.

Arthur: quiet and reserved, prefers privacy. Finds social activities intimidating and stressful.

Elsie: feels isolated and alone. Gets stimulation and satisfaction from contact with others.

In the person's own home

	Integration	*Privacy*
Arthur		
Elsie		

In a residential setting

	Integration	*Privacy*
Arthur		
Elsie		

➡ What were the main differences between Arthur and Elsie?
➡ What were the main differences between the person's home and the residential unit?

Education

A person's educational background is significant when evaluating their performance and abilities. Ngandu *et al.*'s (2007) study highlighted that educated people tend to perform better in dementia screening tests. This might in part be explained by the *cognitive reserve hypothesis* which suggests that highly educated individuals are initially less likely to manifest clinical symptoms of dementia because they are able to use cognitive processing or compensatory approaches to cope better (Roe *et al.* 2007). However, although such people may be able to cope for longer before difficulties are clearly apparent, cognitive decline is usually more rapid following diagnosis due to the increased disease burden (Hall *et al.* 2007). What is apparent here is that some individuals are able to compensate in part for their failing cognitive ability by employing other reserves or strategies. The scores obtained for example on a Mini Mental State Examination (MMSE) test need to be reviewed within a wider context and may differ significantly from person to person with similar levels of cognitive deterioration. We might look at the scenario of conducting MMSE tests with two individuals and find that person A scores significantly higher than person B yet shows a much more marked organic deterioration on their brain scans results. The implications here relate to the need to assess a person and their abilities via a range of different methods and not to be too reliant upon the results of a single test. We might also reflect here upon cognitive strategies that might be taught or facilitated with individuals to help combat memory loss and difficulties in processing information.

Activity 6.4

Can you think of any approaches here which might help individuals who are experiencing problems with:

➡ Forgetfulness?
➡ Confusion?

Dependence/independence

Each person has their own inclination or desire as to whether they would rather look after themselves or seek to be looked after by others. While we might assume that a frail 86-year-old woman entering a nursing home would be only too happy to be taken care of, it might actually be quite destructive for her with her remaining coping skills declining at a faster rate. We can look at all of this in Case Study 6.1 by revisiting Elsie.

Case Study 6.1 Elsie

To recap: Elsie is an 83-year-old widower, who has recently moved into residential care after concerns were raised about her safety and ability to continue living on her own at home. She is a retired veterinarian, and up until recently had kept busy with frequent activities, leisure interests and social engagements. She has fluctuating periods of lucidity and confusion, becoming extremely distressed when aware of what she is not able to do.

Elsie

For most of Elsie's life, she has been the person whom family and friends relied upon. She takes great pleasure in looking after others and seeing things 'done right', and does not like others fussing over her. She takes enormous comfort from the help she can give to other people and her sense of esteem is bolstered by the recognition and gratitude bestowed upon her. Elsie gets very frustrated and upset when confronted by tasks that she is not able to do.

Elsie has recently been admitted to a care home. You notice her get up and try to help lay the table at lunch time although she is clearly struggling and getting upset. She is unable to correctly arrange items on the table and has dropped a significant amount of cutlery onto the floor. She is told not to worry and that others will take care of it *for her*.

Activity 6.5

In response to Case Study 6.1:

➡ How might Elsie feel about this experience?
➡ How could we best respond to this situation?

An assumption commonly made in the care of older people is that of *desired dependence*: a feeling that older people would naturally welcome being looked after. While this may be the case for some people, for others it can spell a huge threat to their fading capabilities and foster feelings such as helplessness. The core issue raised in Activity 6.5 relates to the process whereby individuals are discouraged from using the abilities they have because of the difficulties experienced. Although often done in a paternalistic and caring way or through fears of safety it can severely undermine what is vital to some people: a need to feel useful, competent and purposeful. Taking this away might enhance a person's feelings of helplessness and deny them opportunities to give as well as receive care. This process was recognized by Kitwood (1997) as part of his *enhancing personhood* factors where the person with dementia is able to take the lead role and offer something to their social setting.

Activity 6.6

Tick the box that most applies to the following statements:

	True	False
➡ Old people *like* being looked after	☐	☐
➡ Old people *need* to be looked after	☐	☐
➡ People with dementia *like* being looked after	☐	☐
➡ People with dementia *need* to be looked after	☐	☐
➡ Younger people with dementia are able to look after themselves	☐	☐
➡ Opportunities to be helped are gratefully received	☐	☐
➡ It is too risky to allow those with dementia to do everything they want to	☐	☐
➡ Family carers are especially mindful of promoting independence	☐	☐

What is the rationale for your choices?

Associated health states

> **Activity 6.7**
>
> ➡ What are the different types of dementia?

Type and nature of dementia

The term *dementia* has a number of commonly related assumptions attached to it that can encourage views and expectations about the person and the condition. As diagnoses are more frequently given at a much earlier stage this may apply to individuals whose symptoms seem barely discernible to others. Their presentation might belie the common stereotypical views as they continue to work, drive and socialize, all at high levels of capability. One of the main aspects here relates to the stage of cognitive deterioration a person is experiencing and the specific diagnosis given. There are a number of conditions that fall under the umbrella term of dementia.

Alzheimer's disease

Alzheimer's is the most prevalent type of dementia and is caused by the development of 'plaques' and 'tangles' in the brain. It follows an insidious progress and is marked by confusion, difficulties with memory and language skills, mood swings, behavioural change and a progressive withdrawal of interest.

Vascular dementia

The second most common form of dementia is vascular dementia, caused by problems with the supply of blood to the brain. It is characterized by sudden difficulty with comprehension or carrying out routine tasks, confusion, irritability or aggression, balance and coordination difficulties, difficulties with speech and drowsiness.

Dementia with Lewy bodies (DLB)

This is caused by the presence of protein deposits which disrupt the brain's normal functioning and features problems with confusion, language and memory, hallucinations and delusions, stiffness and tremor, slowness of movement, depression and spatial disorientation

Fronto-temporal dementia (including Pick's disease)

This is caused by damage to the frontal lobe and temporal parts of the brain and features particular characteristics such as personality changes, gluttony and hypersexuality, obsessional behaviour, decreased inhibitions and roaming behaviour.

Other dementias include Korsakoff's syndrome which is associated with heavy drinking over a long period, HIV- and AIDS-related cognitive impairment, particularly in the later stages of a person's illness, and Creutzfeldt-Jakob disease, caused by infectious agents. There are many other rarer causes of dementia, including progressive supranuclear palsy and Binswanger's disease. People with multiple sclerosis, motor neurone disease, Parkinson's disease and Huntington's disease can also be at an increased risk of developing dementia.

Activity 6.8

➡ Which types of dementia have you encountered in practice?
➡ How did the person's presentation of their dementia differ from that of others?

Disability/infirmity

The individual with dementia might also present with various infirmities or types of disability making things such as communication and self-care problematic for them. These problems might be long-standing or have recently developed, due to factors such as old age, illness or trauma – for example, strokes can exacerbate problems with communication (i.e. aphasia/dysphasia where expression of words becomes impaired). As well as verbal content we might also consider the significance and complexity of non-verbal communication including tone and pitch, speed, facial expressions, posture, gestures, paralanguage and eye contact (Morris and Rungapadiachy 2008). Any or all of these can be blocked or compromised through various health deficits.

There are also other age-related features whereby a person's communicative ability is compromised:

- impaired eyesight;
- poor hearing;
- absence of properly fitting dentures.

Physical frailty or disability can also have a significant impact in fostering states of dependency. As well as having to contend with low levels of expectation because of their dementia, any disability or infirmity may further convince others that a person 'needs looking after'. This could relate to a frail nursing home resident who, having fallen on occasions, is thereafter discouraged from moving around independently.

It is also imperative that certain physical problems contributing to confusional states are ruled out, such as infection, constipation, hormonal imbalance or inadequate nutrition (Kitwood 1997).

Associated mental health states

It is important when trying to ascertain signs of deterioration attributable to dementia to be able to rule out effects caused by the presence of coexistent mental health states, primarily those of depression and anxiety but also others such as schizophrenia, bipolar disorder or obsessive compulsive disorder (see Best Fit 6.1 for practice recommendations). Mental health problems might exist independently or develop as a consequence of a person's experience with dementia. Depression, for example, is common in the aftermath of a dementia diagnosis because of its fearful connotations (Kitwood 1997). It is more commonly found in those with dementia than those without (Forsell and Winblad 1998) and is estimated to affect 10–25 per cent of those with Alzheimer's disease (Nilsson *et al.* 2002). The presence of other mental health states can exacerbate or mask symptoms of dementia making accurate assessment difficult, and it might be for example that a person's depressed mood can make their state of cognitive decline appear more pronounced (Insel and Badger 2002). A vivid example of this is provided by Christine Bryden (2005: 17):

> *I had really deteriorated, changing as a person, losing the super-fast, super-smart me. I had become much slower in my speech, less able to make decisions, and more readily confused ... I no longer drove, answered the phone or watched TV, but retreated into gardening and books, as well as early bedtimes.*

From this narrative we might assume that this steady decline is an expected consequence of her Alzheimer's disease. This picture changed though as her mood lifted: 'My head began to clear of the fuzzy "cotton wool" type of feeling that it felt like before. I could concentrate better, and found it easier to speak and listen ... I began to speak on the phone again, and even to start driving again' (Bryden 2005: 18).

The impact that depression has upon a person, such as decreased mood, apathy, poor concentration and withdrawal, might all be easily mistaken as symptoms and signs of cognitive deterioration. It is important therefore to correctly identify and treat underlying depression.

A commonly associated mental health state particularly in mild dementia where insight is retained is that of anxiety disorder (Ballard *et al.* 1994). As highlighted by Shankar and Orrell (2000), it can be difficult to correctly identify because of a fluctuation of symptoms and overlap with features of dementia as well as difficulty for individuals in giving an account of their symptoms. Likewise, anxiety can affect a person in terms of limited social engagement, decreased confidence and lowered performance or involvement with activities as well as a greater propensity for dependency. Anxiety states are often perceived as agitation, a very common expression experienced by around 60 per cent of people with dementia at some stage through their illness (Mintzer and Brawman-Mintzer 1996). A particular problem experienced by those with dementia and expressing agitation concerns the overuse of medication. A study by Ballard *et al.* (2008) found that neuroleptic medication commonly given to agitated Alzheimer's patients makes their condition worse and is associated with a marked deterioration in verbal skills after just six months of treatment. Ballard and Howard (2006) highlight the short-term benefits from neuroleptic use in treating psychiatric and behavioural symptoms but also focus on the serious potential risks which include strokes and increased mortality.

Activity 6.9

Go to your favourite search engine and in the search box type the following terms:

➡ dementia depression;
➡ dementia anxiety.

Best Fit 6.1

• Proper mental health screening should be carried out in order to identify the coexistence of other mental health problems.
• We need to recognize that symptoms of depression and anxiety can be misconstrued as further evidence of cognitive deterioration.
• We should attempt to understand and deal with the *causes* of agitated behaviour. Neuroleptic medication should only be used as a short-term measure with agitation.

Down's syndrome

The clinical picture of Alzheimer's disease in Down's syndrome is complex, owing to the pre-existing cognitive impairment and atypical presentation. Difficulties with making a psychiatric diagnosis in a person with Down's syndrome include 'psychosocial masking', referring to the unsophisticated social skills and lack of life experiences that a person with learning disability might exhibit, thereby altering the presentation of symptoms. Because of their impaired communication skills people with Down's syndrome may not present their symptoms verbally, and it might be left to carers to highlight any changes taking place (Stanton and Coetzee 2004).

There is also the problem posed by 'diagnostic overshadowing' where changes in behaviour or ability are attributed to that person's learning disability (Holland and Benton 2004; Reiss *et al.* 1982). As a consequence, individuals are referred to specialist services late or not at all. Early-onset symptoms may vary from person to person, but there is evidence that the cognitive deficits closely resemble those observed in Alzheimer's disease (Oliver *et al.* 1998). Deterioration in memory, learning and orientation tend to be the first signs, and these symptoms are often accompanied by increased dependence (Cosgrave *et al.* 2000). It has also been reported that Alzheimer's disease in Down's syndrome presents with a greater prevalence of low mood, excessive overactivity, restlessness, disturbed sleep, excessive uncooperativeness and auditory hallucinations (Cooper and Prasher 1998).

A study of 285 people with Down's syndrome found a 13 per cent prevalence of Alzheimer's disease (Tyrell *et al.* 2001). The occurrence of Alzheimer's disease in people with Down's syndrome is regarded as no greater than in the general population although occurring 30–40 years earlier (Holland and Benton 2004). Although the prevalence is found to be rising with increasing age (Visser *et al.* 1997) it is important to recognize that for people with Down's syndrome over the age of 40, decline in functioning is not inevitable (Stanton and Coetzee 2004). This is where low expectations and assumptions again 'take away' many abilities that individuals still retain.

Affiliation

This section looks at the groups a person belongs to by virtue of a number of characteristics including those of:

- culture;
- age;
- gender;
- sexual orientation.

Culture

Dementia as experienced by black and minority ethnic people has become a significant contemporary concern (Yeo and Gallagher-Thompson 1996; Patel *et al.* 1998). Higher incidences of dementia have been found among non-English speaking black and ethnic minority groups although issues of disorientation may be misinterpreted due to language problems (McCracken *et al.* 1997). It is currently estimated that there are approximately 11,500 people in the UK from black and minority ethnic groups with dementia and it is further predicted that the number of people with dementia from this group will rise fairly rapidly, raising concerns about the appropriateness of available resources (Knapp and Prince 2007). These concerns are mirrored in other cultural groups such as the Asian community, where Seabrooke and Milne (2004) report on the poor uptake of healthcare support by people with dementia. Attempts to support these communities have been made with the development of various projects such as the Alzheimer's Society's Black and Minority Ethnic Communities Project. This aimed to increase understanding and share knowledge of dementia by working in partnership with people from the black and minority ethnic communities in London. Another worthy initiative, as illustrated in Box 6.1, was the Meri Yaadain awareness raising and support project (Alzheimer's Society 2008).

Box 6.1 Meri Yaadain

The Bradford-based project Meri Yaadain (*my memories*) is aimed at raising awareness of dementia and providing support for Bradford's South Asian communities. It was found that many people from these communities were not seeking help because they:

- had no concept of dementia;
- thought memory loss was an inevitable consequence of old age;
- were reluctant to seek help because of the stigma attached;
- had a strong sense of family duty to care for older relatives.

An initial problem included working with individuals whose language doesn't contain a word for dementia. The key therefore to the project was linking this condition to memories rather than mental health. Meri Yaadain project workers run roadshows and visit families in their homes offering support and advice and acting as advocates, ensuring that health and social services meet their cultural and language needs.

(Alzheimer's Society *Living Magazine*, September 2008)

Age

The incidence of dementia rises progressively as age advances with the majority of incidences affecting those over 85. There is a current estimate of 700,000 people in the UK with dementia of which 15,000 (2.2 per cent) include young-onset dementia (Alzheimer's Society 2007). It appears that most of the available services and resources are geared towards the older age group and that specific services for young-onset dementia are lacking (Sampson *et al.* 2004). Problems of younger people with dementia have been largely unacknowledged in policy and practice (Tinker 1999). Indeed, Williams *et al.*'s (2001) study reported that the route to specialist services for young people with dementia is uncoordinated and that they encounter a 'pillar to post' process because of difficulties in diagnosis, lack of adequate resources or an unwillingness of some services to take responsibility. High levels of satisfaction were expressed in relation to services provided by the Alzheimer's Society and the specialist early-onset dementia team but difficulties were noted in accessing respite and longer-term care. One example of good practice can be seen at Merevale House, a Warwickshire care home specifically set up for younger people with dementia. This home runs in a more relaxed and informal manner than the traditional care homes approach and aims to keep residents stimulated and active, respecting and maintaining the abilities that they do have and not focusing predominantly on what they cannot do (Alzheimer's Society 2007).

While the symptoms of dementia are similar whatever a person's age, younger people with dementia may have different problems such as:

- being in work at the time of diagnosis;
- having dependent children still living at home;
- having financial commitments;
- being physically fit and behaving in ways that other people find challenging;
- being more aware of their disease in the early stages;
- finding it hard to accept and cope with losing skills at such a young age;
- finding it difficult to access information, support and services for younger people with dementia.

There are some very significant issues here including the heightened impact upon the person and their lifestyle, family dependents, financial commitments and having to give up aspects such as work and driving. While these may also be true of the older person there may be increased difficulties for younger people in terms of acceptance.

Activity 6.10

➡ How would you feel about working with younger people with dementia?
➡ How do their support needs differ from those of older people?
➡ What can be done/offered?

Gender

Although women are deemed to have an increased risk of Alzheimer's (Andersen *et al.* 1999), current figures show a greater prevalence for men within the young-onset group (50–65) yet higher for women with late-onset dementia (Alzheimer's Society 2007). It is unclear as to what exactly the gender differences are concerning the response to dementia and this remains unaddressed to any depth in dementia care research. There is however evidence of gender discrimination (Adams and Clarke 1999) with older women within mental health care facing a system of *double jeopardy* – being exposed to ageist *and* sexist attitudes (Rodeheaver and Datan 1988).

The American Psychiatric Association (2006) reported that the greater life expectancy for women and a tendency to have older partners results in them being more likely to have an adult child as caregiver. As these carers are more likely to have additional responsibilities it often results in an earlier entry into residential care. Various behavioural differences can be observed between the sexes, with males reportedly displaying more aggression (Hall and O'Connor 2004) and sexual expression (Archibald 2002). Given the fact that nursing homes tend to be populated more by female staff and female residents, protective measures might incorporate behavioural and pharmacological interventions which are overly restrictive.

Differences between how men and women adapt to the experience of dementia might relate in part to their previously adopted roles. Factors such as dependence and independence may be significant here, concerned as they are with former financial, social and domestic responsibilities. It is important therefore to look at each person independently and recognize in what ways their former roles have been impacted upon and how best to accommodate these within their current situation – for example, a woman who has derived a core sense of value through caregiving yet now feels useless and unwanted. Kitwood's (1997) *enhancing personhood* approach focuses attention upon ways by which the individual is enabled to still give to others and retain a sense of acceptance and importance.

Sexual orientation

Older people are generally regarded as celibate or asexual, something that has up until recently caused the concept of sexuality to be largely overlooked (Ehrenfeld *et al.* 1999; Archibald 2001). This has led to expressions of sexuality being seen as problems to be managed or treated. These ageist notions are generally coupled with implicit presumptions of heterosexuality and the experience of gay men and lesbians with dementia remains unrecognized, unrecorded and largely ignored from a policy, practice and research perspective (Price 2008). The social discreditation and stigma encountered by gay and lesbian people with mental health problems often results in a concealment of their sexuality to healthcare staff (Meyer 2003). Many older gay men and women may have already lived many years passing themselves off as heterosexual and now find themselves in the very stressful situation of having to share information with healthcare staff yet struggling to remember who knows what and what it might be safe to divulge (Price 2006). This exacerbates the already high levels of anxiety, stress and isolation that are experienced as more situations are perceived as potentially unsafe. One of the respondents in Price's (2006) study of gay carers recounted their experience of having to 'come out' to 12 separate service providers. Other carers noted the embarrassment and distress at having their status and relationship to the person they cared for queried, especially when attempting to access services. The specific experience of lesbians and gay men remains largely invisible and silent with a person's diagnosis of dementia becoming their chief defining characteristic and other social identities being perceived as less important and less pressing.

The way in which gay and heterosexual individuals cope with the effects of dementia could be influenced by their responses to life experiences. The role losses experienced by heterosexuals such as with children leaving home may be different to that of gay individuals. The adoption of flexible gender roles throughout their life span may have allowed the gay man or woman to develop high levels of independence and a positive self-image which help them adjust more positively to the ageing process (Friend 1980). This view is supported by Healey (1994) who highlights that throughout their lifetimes many lesbian women have placed a high premium on their independence and self-reliance, developing 'special and sophisticated strategies' which enable them to survive, including skills that heterosexual women might assign to men. There are a number of implications here including the person's feelings about the sense of *enforced dependency* that is often fostered within residential care.

Activity 6.11

➡ What are the difficulties in practice with ascertaining a person's sexuality/sexual orientation?

➡ Do we try hard enough to help?

➡ What could be done better to make people feel freer to express themselves?

Ascertaining a person's sexual orientation can be for many a problematic and uncomfortable experience. The tendency might be therefore to overlook aspects or to make assumptions based upon the answers given to related questions. As Harrison (2001) suggests, rather than bluntly questioning the other person about their sexuality, we can instead provide spaces, practices, language and symbols that suggest to gay individuals that they are in a non-discriminatory environment, particularly for those who are confused and struggling to find the correct words with which to express themselves.

Losing the *person*

'The Alzheimer face is neither tragic nor comic, as a face can appear in other forms of dementia … The Alzheimer face indicates only an absence: it is a mask in the most literal sense' (Bayley 1999: 59). This sentiment by John Bayley reflects Goldsmith's (1996: 26) findings that: 'In their despair relatives often assert that dementia has destroyed their loved one's personality'. This highlights the general feeling experienced by many relatives and friends of those with dementia – namely that of losing the *person* who is regarded as no longer being there (Kitwood 1997). As the person's ability to communicate diminishes so does the extent to which others are able to recognize and reach the person that resides within. The problem for those with dementia is of having their personhood denied with the assumption that their essential essence has departed.

One of the main requirements within person-centred care is of having the skills, patience and ability to locate the *person* that resides within their condition of dementia. It is a process that can be progressively more difficult as the traces of that individual become obscured by their withdrawal and their deteriorating communicative ability. We must also acknowledge the real personality changes that are attributable to some forms of dementia such as a lessening of inhibitions, which to relatives and friends might present the appearance of a new and different person emerging. While this might include behaviours that seem 'out of character' – for example becoming sexually disinhibited or showing aggressive behaviour – it can also relate to feelings of liberation and enhanced creative expression. What is important perhaps is recognizing that observed changes are not necessarily all representative of further aspects of a person being lost, as it might be that some long-repressed personality characteristics are finally emerging. This relates to Goldsmith's (1996) suggestion of a general continuity of personality in dementia with some characteristics (that were always present) now appearing in an exaggerated form.

Activity 6.12

How much of the problem in locating the *person* within the condition of dementia is down to:

➡ Their inability to express themselves?
➡ Our inability to find them?

Losing the *person* has profound implications for their subsequent care and might influence the ways of working with them, with a greater emphasis upon symptoms and behaviour management. Objectifying the person can lead to some of the negative care approaches identified in Kitwood's (1997) process of *malignant social psychology* (MSP). An example of exploring these factors with students is provided in Exercise 6.1.

Exercise 1: Malignant social psychology (MSP)

This exercise asked healthcare students to consider Kitwood's (1997) MSP factors and how they might be experienced in practice. A full list of these factors and details of this exercise are provided in Chapter 9. Students were asked to consider what causes bad practice approaches to develop and how they might be drawn into these ways of responding. This provoked much discussion and it was noted that while we might distance ourselves from these practices assuming that it is merely 'uncaring' or 'unskilled' staff who respond in these ways, it is important to note that we can easily get drawn into some or all of these responses without even being aware of it. The information provided in Box 6.2 shows some of the justifications which might be given as to why some of the MSP factors are observed.

Box 6.2 MSP factors

MSP factor	Practice problems
Disempowerment – not allowing a person to use the abilities that they do have; failing to help them complete actions they have initiated	*Time constraints* – i.e. 'it's quicker for me to get Elsie dressed than to assist her to do it herself' *Uncaring* – 'it's unkind to stand back and watch people struggle and fail with tasks' *Risk factors* – 'people with dementia are significantly at risk and more prone to harming themselves'
Treachery – using forms of deception in order to distract or manipulate a person or force them into compliance	*External pressures and demands* – 'I will be judged an ineffective practitioner if unable to carry out care interventions' *Internal pressures and demands* – 'I am uncaring if I can't get the patient to take needed medication'
Outpacing – providing information, presenting choices at a rate too fast for a person to understand, putting them under pressure to do things more rapidly than they can bear	*Misreading the other person* – unaware of how the pace of choices given is perceived by the other person *Frustration and impatience* – felt because of other's lack of response, or pressures and demands from others

Objectification – treating a person as if they were a lump of dead matter, to be pushed, lifted, filled, pumped or drained without proper reference to the fact that they are a sentient being	*Inability to see the other person* – more so in late-stage dementia as there is generally a less responsive reaction and a lack of observable cues to help assert sense of personality

Locating the *person*

The essence of good patient care is to reinforce an individual's identity through approaches such as reminiscence work, the composition of life history and life reviews and the use of validation techniques. What we need to recognize here is although some people with dementia may be difficult to find they are still able to engage and relate to external stimuli. It might be simply a smile, a lessening of agitation or sitting more upright and alert that indicates that a person with advanced dementia is able to relate in some meaningful way to their surroundings.

Reminiscence therapy stems from Butler's (1963) work on *life review* in which past experience and unresolved conflicts are brought into a person's consciousness. There are a wide variety of studies that have investigated the value of reminiscence as a therapeutic intervention, and these show marked discrepancies in their definitions of what it is, why it is used and how (Lin *et al.* 2003). It is generally recognized that there are a number of benefits including helping practitioners understand patients more clearly (Clarke *et al.* 2003); helping to create calmness in the present (Rainbow 2003); increasing self-esteem (Finnema *et al.* 2000); improving communication and reinforcing identity (McIntosh and Woodall 1995); and decreasing caregiver strain (Woods *et al.* 2005). The *National Service Framework for Older People* (DoH 2001) Section 1.3 advocates that a person with dementia should be supported in an individualized, sensitive and appropriate way, using their life history to help plan their care and support. However, it is important to note the short-term benefits of life review or reminiscence work which need to be part of a continuous ongoing programme or part of daily activities (Goldwasser *et al.* 1987). Care and consideration need to be shown at all times to the person that reminiscence activities are concerned with sensitivity, appropriateness and interest, thus avoiding the creation of examples such as those illustrated in 'Worst Fit' 6.1.

Worst Fit 6.1

When using reminiscence avoid the following.

- Items that are exclusive and not recognized.
- Distressing or difficult material (e.g. symbols of war).

- Issues that reinforce a person's current plight (in comparison with earlier and better times).
- Predominant focus upon olden days (missing the point that people have also lived through the past few decades).
- Using products or items that people don't like – i.e. 'I hated it then and still do now.'
- Having encouraged emotional responses being unskilled in the distress caused
- Patronizing and dismissive responses to people's reminiscences.

Exercise 2: Planning a reminiscence activity

Healthcare students undertook an exercise to consider the appropriateness of content and process when constructing reminiscence activities to use within practice. Full details are provided in Chapter 9. The task was for students to project themselves 50 years into the future and design a reminiscence activity which they might offer to their peer group. What emerged from this activity was a greater consideration as to what is deemed appropriate as colleagues questioned and challenged the activities planned for them. It was interesting to note the comments of one group member concerning the planned showing of the television programme *Big Brother* as she detested both the show and its presenter. The quality of the feedback and subsequent discussion enabled modifications to be made with further thoughts as to how group activities could be structured to encourage better engagement and interaction.

Enhancing personhood

The issues discussed in this chapter have attempted to understand more about the person we might be working with, thus enabling us to more clearly individualize care. Careful assessment, use of attending skills and involvement of carers helps to build up the picture of who the person before us is, even if their communicative ability has become severely impaired. It enables us to consider some of Kitwood's (1997) *enhancing personhood* factors (see Box 6.3) which relate care approaches more specifically to the person. These can be considered by completing Activity 6.13.

Box 6.3 Enhancing personhood

1 Person with dementia on receiving end
- *Recognition* – acknowledged as a person, affirmed in his/her own uniqueness.
- *Negotiation* – people with dementia are *consulted* as to their preferences, desires and needs.
- *Collaboration* – working together, aligned on a shared task.
- *Play* – spontaneity and self-expression.
- *Timulation* – sensuous or sensual intervention providing contact and pleasure (i.e. aromatherapy).

- *Celebration* – any moment where life is experienced as intrinsically joyful.
- *Relaxation*.
- *Validation* – acknowledging the reality of a person's emotions and feelings.
- *Holding* – providing a safe psychological space.
- *Facilitation* – enabling a person to do what otherwise they would be unable to do.

2 Person with dementia takes lead role
- *Creation* – person with dementia spontaneously offers something to the social setting (i.e. singing or dancing).
- *Giving* – person with dementia expresses concern, affection, gratitude, warmth or sincerity.

Activity 6.13
- Think of a person you are working with at present and consider how the enhancing personhood factors apply to them.

Conclusion

This chapter has considered the person-centred approach with regards to the *person* as a *unified whole*, composed from a myriad of individual personal experiences. This approach regards each person as being different and illustrates why people who share a diagnosis of dementia still require their own individualized care. The importance therefore with person-centred care is to be more mindful as to the make-up and personality of those we are working with and to direct care specifically towards their personal needs as opposed to their assumed or expected needs. This enables us to approach care from a perspective that values and accepts the worth of those we are working with.

Key points
- We need to look at each person as a *unified whole* – composed by their own unique range of experiences. Assumptions therefore should not be based upon our contact with others.
- Person-centred care should be applied to everyone, irrespective of their condition or restrictions with time, staff and resources.
- Person-centred care is not a one-approach-fits-all intervention. It should be adapted to suit the particular needs of those we are working with.
- Person-centred care is essentially concerned with accepting and valuing the worth of the person with dementia.

References

Adams, T. and Clarke, C.L. (eds) (1999) *Dementia Care: Developing Partnerships in Practice*. London: Balliere Tindall.

Alzheimer's Society (2007) *Living with Dementia*, www.alzheimers.org.uk/site/scripts/documents.php?categoryID=200241, accessed 23 September 2008.

Alzheimer's Society (2008) *Living with Dementia*, www.alzheimers.org.uk/site/scripts/documents.php?categoryID=200241, accessed 6 January 2009.

American Psychiatric Association (2006) *Guidelines for the Treatment of Psychiatric Disorders*. Washington, DC: American Psychiatric Publishing.

Andersen, K., Launer, L., Dewey, M., Letenneur, L., Ott, A., Copeland, J., Dartigues, J., Kragh–Sorensen, P., Baldereschi, M., Brayne, C., Lobo, A., Martinez–Lage, J., Stijnen, T. and Hofman, A. (1999) Gender differences in the incidence of AD and vascular dementia: the EURODEM study, *Neurology*, 53(9): 1992–7.

Archibald, C. (2001) Resident sexual expression and the key worker relationship: an unspoken stress in residential care work?, *Practice*, 13(1): 5–12.

Archibald, C. (2002) Sexuality, dementia and residential care: managers report and response, *Health and Social Care in the Community*, 6(2): 95–101.

Ballard, C. and Howard, R. (2006) Neuroleptic drugs in dementia: benefits and harm, *Nature Reviews Neuroscience*, 7: 492–500.

Ballard, C., Mohan, R., Patel, A. and Graham, C. (1994) Anxiety and disorder in dementia, *Irish Journal of Psychological Medicine*, 11(3): 108–9.

Ballard, C., Lana, M., Theodoulou, M., Douglas, S., McShane, R., Jacoby, R., Kossakowski, K., Yu, L. and Juszczak, E. (2008) A randomised, blinded, placebo-controlled trial in dementia patients continuing or stopping neuroleptics (the DART-AD trial), *Nature Clinical Practice: Neurology*, 4(10): 528–9.

Bayley, J. (1999) *Iris: a Memoir of Iris Murdoch*. London: Abacus.

Bryden, C. (2005) *Dancing with Dementia*. London: Jessica Kingsley.

Butler, R. (1963) The life review: an interpretation of reminiscence in the aged, *Psychiatry*, 26: 65–76.

Clarke, A., Hanson, E. and Ross, H. (2003) Seeing the person behind the patient: enhancing the care of older people using a biographical approach, *Journal of Clinical Nursing*, 12: 697–706.

Cooper, S. and Prasher, V. (1998) Maladaptive behaviours and symptoms of dementia in adults with Down's syndrome compared with adults with intellectual disabilities of other aetiologies, *Journal of Intellectual Disability Research*, 42: 293–300.

Cosgrave, M., Tyrrell, J., McCarron, M., Gill, M. and Lawlor, B. (2000) A five year follow-up study of dementia in persons with Down's syndrome: early symptoms and patterns of deterioration, *Irish Journal of Psychological Medicine*, 17: 5–11.

Daker-White, G., Beattie, A., Means, R. and Gilliard, J. (2002) *Serving the Needs of Marginalised Groups in Dementia Care: Younger People and Minority Ethnic Groups. Summary of Key Findings and Conclusions.* Bristol: University of the West of England and Dementia Voice.

DoH (Department of Health) (2001) *National Service Framework for Older People.* London: DoH.

DoH (Department of Health) (2005) *Securing Better Mental Health for Older Adults,* www.dh-.gov.uk, accessed 10 September 2008.

DoH (Department of Health) (2006a) *A New Ambition for Old Age,* www.dh.gov.uk/en/Publicationsandstatistics/Publications/PublicationsPolicyAndGuidance/DH_4133941, accessed 10 September 2008.

DoH (Department of Health) (2006b) *Dignity in Care,* www.dh.gov.uk/en/Policyandguidance/Healthandsocialcaretopics/Socialcare/Dignityincare/index.htm, accessed 10 September 2008.

DoH (Department of Health) (2009) *Living Well with Dementia: A National Dementia Strategy.* London: DoH.

Ehrenfeld, M., Bronner, G., Tabak, N., Alpert, R. and Bergman, R. (1999) Sexuality among institutionalized patients with dementia., *Nursing Ethics,* 6(2): 144–9.

Feil, N. (2002) *The Validation Breakthrough: Simple Techniques for Communicating with People with 'Alzheimer's-Type Dementia',* 2nd edn. Batimore, MD: Health Professions Press.

Finnema, E., Dröes, R., Ribbe, M. and Van Tilburg, W. (2000) The effects of emotion-oriented approaches in the care for persons suffering from dementia: a review of the literature, *International Journal of Geriatric Psychiatry,* 15: 141–61.

Forsell, Y. and Winblad, B. (1998) Major depression in a population of demented and nondemented older people: prevalence and correlates, *Journal of the American Geriatric Society,* 46: 27–30.

Friend, R.A. (1980) 'Gayging: adjustment and the older gay male', *Alternative Lifestyle,* 3(2): 231–48.

Goldsmith, M. (1996) *Hearing the Voice of People with Dementia: Opportunities and Obstacles.* London: Jessica Kingsley.

Goldwasser, A., Auerbach, S. and Harkins, S. (1987) Cognitive, affective and behavioural effects of reminiscence group therapy on demented elderly, *International Journal of Aging and Human Development,* 25(3): 209–22.

Hall, C.B., Derby, C., LeValley, A., Katz, M.J., Verghese, J. and Lipton, R.B. (2007) Education delays accelerated decline on a memory test in persons who develop dementia, *Neurology,* 69(17): 1657–64.

Hall, K. and O'Connor, D. (2004) Correlates of aggressive behaviour, *International Psychogeriatrics,* 16: 141–58.

Harrison, J. (2001) 'It's none of my business': gay and lesbian invisibility in aged care, *Australian Occupational Therapy Journal,* 48: 142–5.

Healey, S. (1994) Diversity with a difference: on being old and lesbian, *Journal of Gay and Lesbian Social Services*, 1(1): 109–17.

Holland, T. and Benton, M. (2004) *Ageing and its Consequences for People with Down's Syndrome. A Guide for Parents and Carers.* Teddington: Down's Syndrome Association.

Insel, K. and Badger, T. (2002) Deciphering the 4 D's: cognitive decline, delirium, depression and dementia – a review, *Journal of Advanced Nursing*, 38(4): 360–8.

King's Fund (1986) *Living Well Into Old Age.* London: King's Fund.

Kitwood, T. (1997) *Dementia Reconsidered.* Maidenhead: Open University Press.

Knapp, M. and Prince, M. (2007) *Dementia UK: The Full Report.* London: Alzheimer's Society.

Lin, Y., Dai, R. and Hwang, S. (2003) The effect of reminiscence on the elderly population: a systemic review, *Public Health Nursing*, 20(4): 297–306.

Maslow, A. (1970) *Motivation and Personality*, 2nd edn. London: Harper & Row.

McCracken, C., Boneham, M., Copeland, K., Williams, K., Wilson, K., Scott, A., McKibbin, P. and Cleave, N. (1997) Prevalence of dementia and depression among elderly people in black and ethnic minorities, *The British Journal of Psychiatry*, 171: 269–73.

McIntosh, I.B. and Woodall, K. (1995) *Dementia: Management for Nurses and Community Care Workers.* London: Quay Books.

Meyer, I. (2003) Prejudice, social stress, and mental health in lesbian, gay and bisexual populations: conceptual issues and research evidence, *Psychological Bulletin*, 129(5): 674–97.

Mintzer, J. and Brawman-Mintzer, O. (1996) Agitation as possible expression of generalised anxiety disorder in demented elderly patients: towards a treatment approach, *Journal of Clinical Psychiatry*, 57: 55–63.

Moos, R. and Lemke, S. (1985) Specialised living environments for older people, in J. Birren and K. Schaie (eds) *Handbook of the Psychology of Aging.* New York: Reinhold.

Morris, J. and Rungapadiachy, D. (2008) Interpersonal communication and interpersonal skills, in D. Rungapadiachy (ed.) *Self Awareness in Health Care.* Basingstoke: Palgrave Macmillan.

Ngandu, T., von Strauss, E., Helkala, E., Winblad, B., Nissinen, A., Tuomilehto, J., Soininen, H. and Kivipelto, M. (2007) Education and dementia: what lies behind the association?, *Neurology*, 69(14): 1442–50.

Nilsson, F., Kessing, L., Sørensen, T., Andersen, P. and Bolwig, T. (2002) Enduring increased risk of developing depression and mania in patients with dementia, *Journal of Neurology, Neurosurgery and Psychiatry*, 73(1): 40–4.

Oliver, C., Crayton, L., Holland, A., Hall, S. and Bradbury, J. (1998) A four year prospective study of age-related cognitive change in adults with Down's syndrome, *Psychological Medicine*, 28: 1365–77.

Patel, N., Mirza, N.R., Lindblad, P. and Samaoli, O. (1998) *Dementia and Minority Ethnic Older People: Managing Care in the UK, Denmark and France.* Lyme Regis: Russell House.

Price, E. (2006) Ageing against the grain: gay men and lesbians, in P. Burke and J. Parker (eds) *Social Work and Disadvantage: Addressing Issues of Stigma through Association*. London: Jessica Kingsley.

Price, E. (2008) Pride or prejudice? Gay men, lesbians and dementia, *British Journal of Social Work*, 38(7): 1337–52.

Rainbow, A. (2003) *The Reminiscence Skills Training Handbook*. Milton Keynes: Speechmark Publishing.

Rodeheaver, D. and Datan, N. (1988) The challenge of double jeopardy – towards a mental health agenda for aging, *American Psychologist*, 43(8): 648–54.

Roe, C., Xiong, C., Miller, H., Phillip, A. and Morris, J. (2007) Education and Alzheimer disease without dementia: support for the cognitive reserve hypothesis, *Neurology*, 68(3): 223–8.

Rogers, C. (1961) *On Becoming a Person: A Therapist's View of Psychotherapy*. Boston, MA: Houghton Mifflin.

Sampson, E., Warren, J. and Rossor, M. (2004) Young onset dementia, *Postgraduate Medical Journal*, 80: 125–39.

Seabrooke, V. and Milne, A. (2004) What will people think? Why is it that elderly Asian people are not accessing dementia services, despite evident need?, *Mental Health Today*, April: 27–30.

Shankar, K. and Orrell, M. (2000) Detecting and managing depression and anxiety in people with dementia, *Current Opinion in Psychiatry*, 13(1): 55–9.

Stanton, L. and Coetzee, R. (2004) Down's syndrome and dementia, *Advances in Psychiatric Treatment*, 10: 50–8.

Tinker, A. (1999) *Younger People with Dementia: Planning, Practice and Development*. London: Jessica Kingsley.

Tyrell, J., Cosgrave, M., McCarron, M., McPherson, J., Calvert, J., Kelly, A., McLaughlin, M., Gill, M. and Lawlor, B.A. (2001) Dementia in people with Down's syndrome, *International Journal of Geriatric Psychiatry*, 16: 1168–74.

Visser, F., Aldenkamp, A., Van Huffelen, A., Van Killman, M., Overweg, J. and van Wijk, J. (1997) Prospective study of the prevalence of Alzheimer type dementia in institutionalized individuals with Down syndrome, *American Journal on Mental Retardation*, 101: 400–12.

Williams, T., Cameron, I. and Dearden, T. (2001) From pillar to post – a study of younger people with dementia, *Psychiatric Bulletin*, 25: 384–7.

Woods, B., Spector, A., Jones, C., Orrell, M. and Davies, S. (2005) *Reminiscence therapy for dementia (Cochrane Review)*, *The Cochrane Library*, 4 (2006).

Yeo, G. and Gallagher-Thompson, D. (1996) *Ethnicity and the Dementias*. Washington, DC: Taylor & Francis.

Further reading

Alzheimer's Disease International (2007). *Younger People With Dementia*, www.alz.co.uk/, accessed 25 June 2008.

Buckwalter, J., Rizzo, A., McCleary, R., Shankle, D., Dick, M. and Henderson, V. (1996) Gender comparisons of cognitive performances among vascular dementia, Alzheimer disease, and older adults without dementia, *Archives of Neurology*, 53(5): 436–9.

Clarke, C. (1999) Partnerships in dementia care: taking it forward, in T. Adams and C. Clarke (eds) *Dementia Care: Developing Partnerships in Practice*. London: Bailliere Tindall.

Draper, B., Moore, C. and Brodarty, H. (1998) Suicidal ideation and the 'wish to die' in dementia patients: the role of depression, *Age and Ageing*, 27: 503–7.

Lindesay, J. and Skea, D. (1997) Gender and interactions between care staff and elderly nursing home residents with dementia, *International Journal of Geriatric Psychiatry*, 12(3): 344–8.

Perrault, A., Wolfson, C., Egan, M., Rockwood, K. and Hogan, D. (2002) Prognostic factors for functional independence in older adults with mild dementia: results from the Canadian study of health and aging, *Alzheimer Disease and Associated Disorders*, 16(4): 239–47.

Proctor, G. (2001) Listening to older women with dementia: relationships, voices and power, *Disability and Society*, 16(3): 361–76.

Reiss, S., Levitan, G.W. and Szyszko, J. (1982) Emotional disturbance and mental retardation: diagnostic overshadowing, *American Journal of Mental Deficiency*, 86: 567–74.

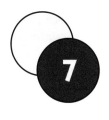

7 Engagement: connecting with the *person*

Objectives: After reading this chapter you should be able to:

➡ Reflect upon the obstacles and difficulties encountered when attempting to engage with those experiencing dementia.

➡ Discuss some of the strategies and interventions which help to connect us with those we are working with.

➡ Explore what engagement means and why it is so important to those with dementia.

Clinical problems (the person with dementia's perspective)

'I can't get on with Arthur, it's simply a clash of personalities.'

'I knew Elsie was upset and I put my hand on her arm but she shrugged it off and didn't seem to want my help.'

'The individuals I work with are simply too confused to be able to engage with. We need to content ourselves instead with giving the best physical care possible.'

And yet … engagement is vital in order to limit the degree of detachment and isolation felt by those with dementia within what they perceive to be an ever-shrinking world.

Introduction

This chapter is about the different types of interaction that occur between health carers and those experiencing dementia. As will be highlighted below, it essentially addresses the process of engagement whereby information moves in a cyclical manner between the two parties concerned. This process can be mutually satisfying or alternatively frustrating as various obstacles and difficulties are encountered. For the purposes of this chapter, the term *engagement* can be defined as the process of making a connection with the inner world of another person. It involves having an awareness and appreciation of their felt experiences and the appropriate skills to relay something of our understanding back to them. As illustrated by Figure 7.1 the process of engagement needs to be seen as two-way and requires understanding to be conveyed back – thereby enabling the other person to feel heard, accepted and valued. The essence of this is a process of reaching out to another human being and enabling them to share with the sense of connectedness. Therefore, it is not enough for me to talk about being empathic because I feel I understand another person, but is something that needs to be acknowledged and felt by *them*.

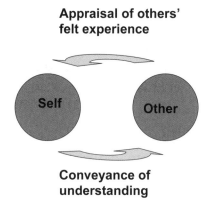

Appraisal of others' felt experience

Self   **Other**

Conveyance of understanding

Figure 7.1 Connecting with others

Activity 7.1

Reflect upon individuals with dementia you work with and consider how many of them you feel you get on with or understand.

➡ What do you feel helps?
➡ What do you feel hinders this process?

There are a number of factors which can positively or negatively influence the engagement process. These include characteristics relating to the person with dementia, the healthcare practitioner or the environment where care takes place. The deteriorating level of cognition and expressive abilities places special demands upon the healthcare practitioner especially when moderate to later stage dementia is experienced as interpretations can become confusing and difficult to comprehend. Of major significance concerning the work with people experiencing dementia is the ability to develop and utilize higher-order communication skills which enable a connection to be made with their experience, thoughts and feelings. It is an approach that has been explored and focused upon in some detail with regards to healthcare practice and in particular can be related to concepts such as validation and empathy.

The difficulties experienced with engagement need not necessarily be related to a person's cognitive deficits as other influencing factors may be present. While we feel quickly drawn towards some people and enjoy the process of getting to know them and working with them, others we struggle with and find contact awkward and uncomfortable. In some circumstances relationship difficulties may be heightened by what is not known about the other person, raising questions as to how much we properly appreciate them. Information can be obtained from:

- the person with dementia;
- family and friends;
- other healthcare workers;
- care plans and professional notes;
- personal observation.

We need to piece all of these written, oral and visual observations together in order to appreciate and get a sense of this other person. As with Gestalt theory, it is the unified 'whole' (*the whole is more than the sum of its parts*) that is important (King and Wertheimer 2005). This relates to the process of perceiving and integrating various snippets of information and attempting to come up with a correct understanding. Obviously, some aspects might be well-documented or 'known' by the healthcare team and corroborated by various sources, such as the statement 'Elsie enjoys drawing'. Knowing about a person's previous occupation, hobbies/interests or family life helps, although it only gives us an idea and not the total picture. Because Elsie at one point in her life enjoyed drawing doesn't mean that we should engage her in this activity without attempting to ascertain her current feelings. It might be that Elsie now finds drawing extremely frustrating and lacking in enjoyment because of fading eyesight, arthritic joints and poor concentration. Engagement is therefore much more than simply *knowing* about another person. It entails a felt component whereby what is going on internally for them is also grasped and related to by the healthcare practitioner.

The person with dementia may experience many significant emotions and thoughts that have a strong bearing on their subsequent behaviour. For example, a recalled family outing might instigate a feeling of calmness and pleasure. By contrast, a confused remonstration from a fellow resident might make that person feel threatened and uncomfortable. The issue here is to what extent this individual is able to share or express these feelings. The former example relates to one of the features Kitwood (1997) identified as helping to enhance personhood – that of *celebration*, a moment where life is experienced as intrinsically joyful, while the latter example alerts us to the potential difficulties in correctly interpreting a person's behaviour: without prior knowledge of the precursor, we are liable to respond incorrectly and perhaps enforce boundaries rather than offer supportive guidance. Properly engaging with another person means gaining an appreciation of their underlying emotions and feelings, thereby reducing the potential for misinterpretation where underlying issues and feelings are missed.

Activity 7.2

Think about individuals with dementia whom you never really get to know or whose company you don't particularly enjoy.

➡ What has influenced this situation?
➡ How could it be improved?

Why is engagement important?

Activity 7.3

➡ Briefly consider what you feel to be the potential benefits from the process of engagement.

Benefits for the carer are . . .

Benefits for the person experiencing dementia are . . .

....

....

....

....

....

....

As Activity 7.3 explored, there are a number of benefits to be had for both parties when feeling more connected. Healthcare staff have reported feeling more motivated and better predisposed to those they are working with when understanding more of the person residing within the condition of dementia. The benefits for the person with dementia are of boosting their self-esteem, feeling more valued and acknowledged and less isolated. Further recommendations for practice are provided in Best Fit 7.1.

Best Fit 7.1

The importance of engaging with those experiencing dementia cannot be overemphasized because of what it offers to both parties involved. The most significant aspects can be regarded as:

• lessening of isolation;
• connecting with the person and not their condition;
• motivating and improving the carer's attitude;
• a mutually satisfying and enjoyable process.

Isolation

The problem of social isolation among those experiencing mental health problems is a significant one and has been well documented by a variety of agencies (DoH 2001, 2006, 2009). The Social Exclusion Unit in their document *Participation in Action on Mental Health – A Guide to Promoting Social Inclusion* includes the statement that: 'Mental ill health does contribute to social exclusion because it affects your confidence to participate in the life of your community' (DoH 2006: 20). Although 'mental ill health' covers a vast range of conditions, this can clearly be applied to those experiencing dementia who are faced with varying levels of cognitive impairment and a growing sense of isolation and helplessness. Feelings of detachment can be seen with the steady erosion of familiar 'landmarks' which help individuals to orientate to and make sense of the world around them. As their condition deteriorates they are left with the sensation and experience of a progressively shrinking world. Some of the commonly experienced dynamics include a growing sense of alienation, disorientation and isolation. This is borne out by Perrin's (1997) study which utilized a dementia care mapping approach with nine clinical settings, finding that individuals with severe dementia were significantly deprived of human contact and that much of that contact was superficial or brief. One could at this point consider the impact that this is likely to have upon a person's concept of self and their methods of coping. We perhaps take for granted aspects or needs that are normally satisfied on a regular basis through interaction with others and our ability to be cognizant of ongoing experiences. For the person experiencing dementia there are numerous reasons to suggest that their perception and feelings about everyday events are being affected in ways that sharply contrast with a young child's attempts to make sense of the world around them. Instead of the growing confidence and sense of awareness attained by the child, the person with dementia is faced with things becoming *less* familiar and *less* understandable. The sense of growing wonder and excitement (felt through the early years) are replaced with trepidation and uncertainty. This generates urges such as the desire to withdraw and retreat away to a place of safety. It is obviously a very solitary and lonely place where we might assume that there is a strong need to share and connect with others. The problem here for carers is perhaps in overlooking what the full impact of this experience might be. Assumptions that simply being with others and joining in with shared activities might meet this need fail to acknowledge the totality of this experience and the impact that it has. While to some degree addressing the need for *inclusion* as advocated by Maslow (1970) and Kitwood (1997), the importance for the person experiencing dementia is in feeling a sense of connection through multi-faceted means – including emotional and psychological channels. The value of engagement can certainly be highlighted through recognizing the detrimental effects that disengagement has upon a person and the resultant experience of social exclusion.

Activity 7.4

➡ Have a look at Robert Davis's (1989) *My Journey into Alzheimer's Disease* and his account of his condition which includes a fluctuating sense of detachment.

Understanding behaviour

The need to properly interpret the behaviour of others is highlighted by the third of Naomi Feil's (1993: 29) *ten key principles of validation* which states: 'There is a reason behind the behaviour of disoriented old-old people'. It is not always easy for healthcare practitioners to correctly identify what a person's observed behaviour might denote, especially if their ability to communicate becomes significantly impaired. We can easily fail to understand what another person might be experiencing and deal with their observed behaviour over that of their felt need. For example, we might act quickly to subdue and quieten down a person who is shouting and wishing to leave the healthcare area instead of dealing with that individual's sense of frustration and need – perhaps to simply have some quiet time walking in the grounds. Understanding another's behaviour involves gaining an appreciation of their underlying emotions which allows us to redefine that person's actions through an awareness of the wider context. It can be seen, for example, with reframing the *sexually disinhibited* individual as somebody seeking and in need of closeness and intimacy. The need therefore is, through engagement, to see beyond the observed behaviour and place it, no matter how bizarre, confusing or disagreeable it appears, into its proper context.

As Killick and Allan (2001) stress, we need to remind ourselves that each person was unique before developing dementia and that we should not assume that all of their subsequent behaviour is necessarily connected with this condition. For example, a person who says very little and keeps their head down might always have been a quiet, withdrawn person. Likewise, someone who's speech is loud and forceful might have been an extroverted type of person all their life. The challenge therefore is to remain open-minded and maintain a questioning approach to what we perceive from the other person. As Kitwood (1997) stresses, it also involves a process of *recognition*, keeping an open and unprejudiced attitude, free from tendencies to stereotype. As much of this might be unconscious on our part, the value of clinical supervision and opportunities to discuss our approach with others is underlined.

Healthcarers' attitudes

As strongly highlighted by Feil (1993), all people are valuable and unique regardless of how disoriented they might be. This person-centred philosophy is reflected through the approach of *personhood* as advocated by Tom Kitwood and the Bradford Dementia Group (Kitwood 1997). Connecting and engaging with a person helps the carer in relating *person to person* rather than *person to condition*. The more that carers are reminded that there is a unique and sentient being before them, regardless of whatever degree of infirmity they encounter, the greater the benefits are for both parties. Some of the benefits for the carer are illustrated by Zimmerman *et al.*'s (2005) study which found that the utilization of person-centred approaches to dementia care resulted in enhanced job satisfaction and personal well-being. This means that there is a gain for both parties as feeling good about the care we give promotes personal feelings of worth and self-esteem. This challenges some of the practices which may arise without one realizing it. For example, Phair and Good

(1995) observed the process of communication by carers as being mainly giving instructions and collecting information but not including conversations. This partly arises from ageist attitudes or an undervaluing of those with dementia with assumptions that gravitate around 'they won't remember facts or understand what is being said'. The process of engagement challenges this by placing the focus firmly back onto the person with dementia. It reminds us who this process of communication is mainly about. We might not get the expected approval or gratification from conversations with individuals experiencing dementia but we can gain a lot from the sense of making a difference for the person we are with. A simple smile, a brief shared recollection or the time spent with another human being may seem fairly small to us as we move onto providing care to someone else, but for the individual concerned it can be of immense value. The impression gained by them might be of being *worth* spending time with. Self-esteem needs, and inclusion needs, are therefore promoted.

Influences on engagement

There are a number of factors which influence the process of engagement, either enabling or obstructing this process (see Figure 7.2). These factors can be seen as relating to three core aspects, namely those of:

- *self* (the healthcare worker);
- *person with dementia*;
- *environment* (location where care takes place).

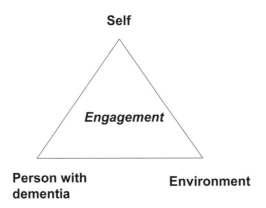

Figure 7.2   Engagement

Exercise 1: Three circles

The three circles exercise was used with healthcare students (see Chapter 9 for full details) and looks at how our degree of engagement alters according to the other person's condition. Essentially, this exercise looks at the extent to which we recognize certain components (P, the person and D, the condition of dementia) as relating to those we are working with. It highlights some of the problems faced in practice when the *condition of dementia* starts to become much more visible than the *person*. It was evident from students that the component of *dementia* was related to much more strongly than that of the *person* within residential or later-stage dementia care settings, although the opposite was found for those in earlier stages or still residing in their own homes. Some of the most important factors were felt to be the person's communicative and expressive ability as well as the range of reinforcing cues accessible – i.e. pictures, possessions or other family members. The need within care approaches is to use interventions and approaches that create a better balance, being less about the condition of dementia and more about the person with dementia.

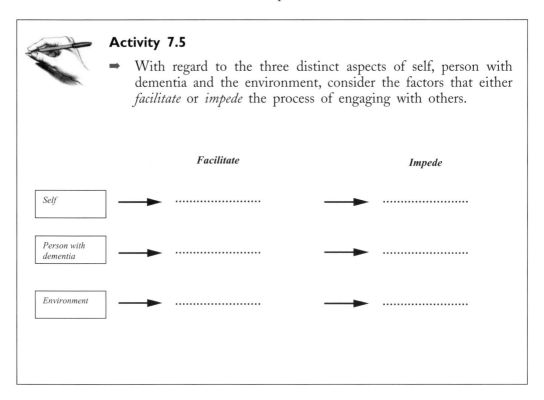

Activity 7.5

➡ With regard to the three distinct aspects of self, person with dementia and the environment, consider the factors that either *facilitate* or *impede* the process of engaging with others.

	Facilitate	*Impede*
Self	....	....
Person with dementia	....	....
Environment	....	....

Self

A number of issues will clearly influence the ability of carers to connect with those they are caring for. The first component to be considered concerns that of self and the ways in which certain aspects might impact upon your ability to engage with others. Of prime importance here is the degree of self-awareness that is held by carers, particularly in relation to the various factors that help them get closer to another's experience or conversely cause them to move away. Certainly within dementia care, as with any other clinical speciality, there are elements within our conscious and unconscious awareness that play a fundamental part in how we relate to others. One way of looking at this is through Luft and Ingram's (1955) concept of the Johari Window (see Figure 7.3) which illustrates the distinction between different aspects of self that are known to us and others. As highlighted in quadrant 2, there are *blind* areas, factors not known to us, yet observable by others. For example, we may through clinical supervision become aware of aspects previously not realized by us such as our *favouring* of certain individuals who make us feel needed.

	Known to self	*Not known to self*
Known to others	**Open**	**Blind**
Not known to others	**Hidden**	**Unknown**

Figure 7.3   The Johari Window

Furthermore, O'Connor and Seymour's (1990) illustration of the dynamics between a person's *internal response* and *external behaviour* helps to reveal the interpersonal processes operating between two people (see Figure 7.4).

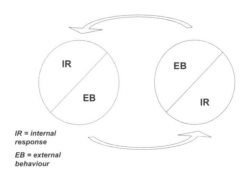

IR = internal
response

EB = external
behaviour

Figure 7.4   Internal response/external behaviour

As this model demonstrates, the relationship between the two parties is reliant upon subsequent interpretations of each other's behaviour. It is not simply down to the perception of how others present themselves but is also strongly concerned with the feelings evoked. This is illustrated by Case Study 7.1 which highlights that the carer needs to be aware of how the other person's behaviour makes them feel and their subsequent reaction, be it of a connecting or distancing nature. It means being aware of the various issues that draw us towards individuals whom we want to spend time with or alternatively maintain a distance from. Another aspect worth considering here is the way in which a person's particular make-up influences the ways by which they interpret incoming stimuli. Through this example we might consider the understanding that is formed by channelling data through a particular frame of reference. This obviously affects the process of engagement and raises the question as to whether one has effectively connected with the other person.

Case Study 7.1 Elsie

To recap: Elsie is an 83-year-old woman living in a residential mental health unit. She is a widower, her husband Sidney having died ten years ago. Elsie has fluctuating periods of lucidity and confusion and is rarely visited by family or friends.

Elsie

Elsie feels lost and scared (*internal response*) and is currently looking for her husband to console and support her. She is becoming increasingly frustrated and angry with her inability to locate him and has started shouting and pushing people away in her agitation and confusion (*external behaviour*). The carer is unaware as to the cause of this although is very aware of how Elsie's behaviour makes him feel – intimidated and threatened (*internal response*). This evokes a reaction in the carer where his subsequent reaction is predominantly defensive and attempting to retain control (*external behaviour*). This approach comes across to Elsie as dismissive and unsupportive, making her feel vulnerable and unsure (*internal response*), thereby generating a whole new cycle of dynamics.

The person with dementia

The particular problems for engagement located within the person with dementia relate largely to a declining communicative ability. Some of the language difficulties experienced by those with dementia are illustrated by Hamdy (1998) as:

- *anomia* – inability to find the right word; a patient in the early stages might use other words to describe objects;

- *agnosia* – in addition to not being able to name an object the patient is also unable to identify what an object is or what it is used for; this can relate to people as well and there may be difficulties in recognizing family members;
- *aphasia* – inability to communicate needs or understand what one hears, including
  - *echolalia* – repetition of words and questions
  - *paralalia* – a single word is repeated again and again
  - *logoconia* – the first syllable is repeated again and again
  - *mutism* – complete absence of speech;
- *apraxia of speech* – difficulty planning the movements necessary for speech;
- *dysarthria* – difficulty in articulation as certain speech sub-systems (i.e. respiration, phonation, resonance and movements of jaw and tongue) are affected.

Recognizing and working with the limitations caused by dementia is vital and perhaps we can regard the restrictive types of expression almost as a unique language in its own right – *the language of dementia*. It means having to open ourselves up to new learning and attempting to understand what a person is communicating to us when words begin to lose their potency. In order to do this we need to tune ourselves in to other aspects of that person's communication such as body language, intonation, expressive gestures or facial expressions. Although these elements are present in each communication, they form to some degree the unnoticed aspects as a large proportion of our attention is taken up by the verbal content of a person's communication.

With the communicative difficulties expressed above it is perhaps understandable that spontaneous speech deteriorates. This does not take account of other complementary features such as a person's anxiety level, absence of dentures or presence of a stammer (which they may incidentally have had prior to developing dementia). As a person's impairment increases it will be harder to concentrate and their speech will become less coherent. Words and themes from previous conversations may intrude in the present and individuals might be hampered by an inability to find the correct terms for what they are trying to express. Obviously, carers need to show understanding and a great deal of patience as simple communication becomes an extremely arduous and frustrating process.

What struck us when working with healthcare students was the frequently reported difficulties in engaging with others or offering choice because of the inability of the other person to respond or properly articulate their thoughts and feelings. Because students or others in their current care settings could not understand what the person was requesting, choices were often then made on their behalf. This problem clearly affects many carers across a wide variety of dementia care settings. We need to look closely at how we respond when faced with patients who are finding it difficult to articulate their needs or wishes. There are often *reasons* cited as to why we take over and decide what those with dementia want, such as:

- 'we don't have enough time';
- 'the person with dementia is too confused to understand what they are being asked';
- 'we're understaffed – I've lots of other people to attend to'.

Or perhaps simply the belief that the carer knows best.

These reported problems provided the impetus for the development of an experiential teaching exercise – *the language of dementia* (full details provided in Chapter 9). This exercise was aimed at helping develop more creative and thoughtful responses when interacting with individuals who have an impaired expressive ability.

Exercise 2: The language of dementia

We first asked students to let us know who had a passing knowledge in any language other than English. Had this not applied then a written list of items in another language (i.e. French) could have been given to read from. The task here was for participants to take on the role of individuals with dementia and express their choices in a language that was incomprehensible to their listeners. This concerned what they wanted:

- to wear;
- eat for breakfast;
- do as an activity.

Other roles were assigned to the remaining students as 'carers' and clinical supervisors. The main issue for carers was to try and ascertain what the other person was trying to communicate by becoming more creative and thoughtful in their use of resources (i.e. pictures and objects) or their reading of the other person's total communication such as vocal characteristics, gestures, signs and facial expressions. What became clear from this exercise was our general reliance upon words and our lack of inventiveness when it comes to 'tuning in' to the total expression of another person. The need is to consider the multitude of other ways that we can reinforce or amplify the 'unnoticed' messages being sent out. It means trying to engage with the other person in a way which is meaningful and allowing for connections to be made. In our impatience or helplessness we perhaps give up all too easily with the assumption that the other person cannot be reached or understood.

Clearly, the methods highlighted above provide carers with ways of understanding the other person's experience and of being able to convey messages back to them. It is the encouragement of a two-way process of communication that is important and not the typical one-way approach which was observed by Goldsmith (1996) whereby the difficulty in comprehending the other person leads to the carer not waiting for a response, or alternatively providing a response for them. Recommendations for practice are provided in Best Fit 7.2.

Activity 7.6

➡ Have a look at Chapter 4, 'Language' in Killick and Allan's (2001) *Communication and the Care of People with Dementia.*

Best Fit 7.2

Develop a repertoire of approaches/modes with which to promote communication including:

- pictures;
- cue cards;
- exaggerated gestures and facial expressions;
- drawing;
- singing;
- dancing.

Environment

The environment within which a person is cared for presents different influences affecting the ability of the carer and the person experiencing dementia to engage with each other. The types of setting can be categorized as:

- own home;
- daycare facility;
- residential healthcare facility.

Activity 7.7

➡ What do you think might help or hinder the process of engagement concerning these different settings?

	Helps	Hinders
Own home	....	....
	....	....
Daycare facility	....	....
	....	....
Residential healthcare facility	....	....
	....	....

The person's own home in many cases offers much richness and multiple cues for engagement. As you gaze around a person's living space you are offered glimpses of their life with information that may be otherwise unattainable within a healthcare setting. The objects and layout of the premises tell us much about the other person and allow us to make inferences about what is important for them. What we have here is a mine of information that can inform us about the other person, most of which may be lost or absent if meeting the person outside this setting. Case Study 7.2 provides an example of what might be picked up when visiting a person's house.

Case Study 7.2 Arthur

To recap: Arthur is a 55-year-old gentleman with vascular dementia. He is married with three grown-up children. He has few hobbies or outside interests as large amounts of his time were taken up through his previous occupation (manager of a small haulage company). He has poor short-term memory although he still retains a good awareness of past events. A significant number of day-to-day experiences are confusing for him and cause impatience and frustration.

Arthur

On entering Arthur's house the first thing I notice is the large number of antiques on show. These fit tastefully within the house itself which is a converted barn with many natural features exposed. There are a lot of photographs on the walls including one of a rugby team holding up a trophy (I notice a player in the front row who bears a strong resemblance to Arthur – although presumably taken many years ago). A number of other photos seem to be of family outings with seaside, mountain and forest scenery. The shelves are filled with books and videos. I can pick out a number of classics and detective novels among the books while comedy and period drama predominate among the videos. On the table are a number of fishing magazines and behind it a dog basket which on this occasion is occupied by a golden retriever.

While the above information need not necessarily relate to Arthur himself it does provide us with a valuable starting point from which to learn about his life. There is a chance that the books and videos do not belong to Arthur, that he rarely reads or watches television, and has a loathing of fishing – 'completely pointless activity' – and that he barely tolerates the dog, especially as his shoes and slippers are frequently chewed up. We do however have a starting point, things that we can check out and discuss with him and his family.

What is especially important about a person's home setting is the presence of opportunities to maintain valued skills, hobbies and interests – for example, the proximity of books, DVDs and CDs. Being in one's own space provides the stimulus for looking after personal needs and wishes. Within the healthcare facility we find it harder to match these opportunities although some daycare provision is more geared up to this because of the emphasis placed upon social and occupational care. It is also worth noting the detrimental impact often found for people entering long-term residential care (Goffman 1961; Moos and Lemke 1985; Perrin 1997). This reflects Lawton and Nahemow's (1973) *environment docility hypothesis* whereby individuals may not engage in previously favoured activities even though they retain the necessary abilities. There are a number of other core factors with regard to the social milieu that include restrictions in time, resources and staffing levels as well as the overall climate of care (degree to which the culture and healthcare team foster and encourage person-centred approaches).

Empathy and validation

The process of engagement involves the ability of the carer to accurately 'tune in' to another's world and communicate this understanding back to them. The essence of this process has been well documented with regards to the therapeutic relationship and may be reflected through terms such as *empathy* or *validation*. We can begin by looking at the process of empathy and consider its definition by Carl Rogers as: 'To sense the client's private world as if it were your own' (1961: 284). Truax (1961) adds to this with the view that it also involves the therapist's verbal facility to communicate their understanding back to the client in a language that is attuned to that person's feelings. Another element, as highlighted by Cassedy and Cutliffe (1998), relates to an affective component which is concerned with helpers caring for their clients. These statements highlight the importance of not only gaining an awareness and appreciation of how things seem from another's vantage point but also being able to convey our understanding back to them. It is about a two-way flow of communication and depends upon each party being able to effectively transmit and receive information. We can consider here the potential obstacles posed when working with those experiencing dementia. Obviously, the extent of a person's cognitive deficiency will play a large part in this process as an impaired ability to verbalize and express one's feelings as well as to comprehend what is fed back will affect the extent of engagement possible. There are also potential problems here for the carer as the extreme nature of a person's distress can cause them to psychologically move away from the other person (Gladstein 1983). For example, one might pick up on the extreme sense of despair acknowledged by someone who is expressing suicidal ideation as a consequence of their awareness of fading cognition and abilities. This can be extremely unsettling and upsetting for the carer who is brought into connection with levels of distress and suffering they might not be able to cope with and therefore might evoke a reassuring or distracting response from them as a means of coping.

A related term to that of empathy is that of validation, an approach that is seen by Feil (1993) as providing disoriented old people with an empathetic listener, someone who accepts and does not judge their view of reality. The validation approach is based on a set of underlying principles that essentially focus upon the uniqueness and value inherent in each person. It is about communicating acceptance to the other person and recognizing that there is a reason for all behaviour exhibited. It also stresses that, through allowing painful feelings to be expressed and acknowledged, they will diminish, but if ignored or suppressed they will gain strength. A number of aspects highlighted here are important with regard to the process of engagement – for example, the acknowledgement that all behaviour has a reason is extremely significant as relating to the carer's attitude to the other person. We might consider here the overworked care staff member who is tiring of a person with dementia's repetitive 'demands' and (along with other staff) labels them as an 'attention seeker'. This obviously addresses the care worker's immediate feelings of frustration and irritation but does very little to address the actual processes and dynamics occurring, namely another individual seeking affection and company from another person. Practice recommendations are provided in Best Fit 7.3.

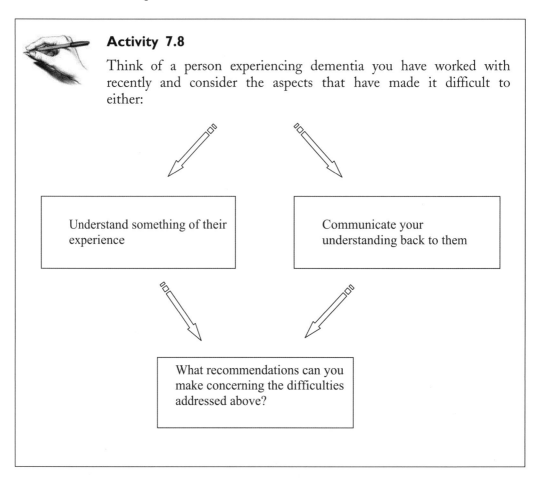

Activity 7.8

Think of a person experiencing dementia you have worked with recently and consider the aspects that have made it difficult to either:

Understand something of their experience

Communicate your understanding back to them

What recommendations can you make concerning the difficulties addressed above?

Best Fit 7.3 Developing an empathic approach

When attempting to develop empathic approaches you need to recognize:

- how much distress you feel comfortable with;
- how you respond to or engage with difficult feelings (i.e. with a rescuing or avoiding approach);
- the tendency to offer reassurance too quickly;
- what you are able to convey of your understanding back to the other person.

The need to connect with those experiencing dementia is important as our knowledge and understanding as to what is really happening to those affected is still very basic (Goldsmith 1996). There is almost a sense of mystery about the person's inner world and Jacques (1992) questions whether the 'previous' person has disappeared or 'unbecome'. Obviously, views concerning what has happened to the person within the condition of dementia fuel different approaches (including negative frameworks) such as that of *objectification*, one of Kitwood's (1997) malignant social psychology factors. Clearly, the greater the level of a person's cognitive impairment, the harder it will be for carers to connect and understand, which perhaps highlights a need to try at earlier stages when it is still possible (Jacques 1992). It is perhaps also down to the carer's attitude as we might reach a stage when we stop trying to reach another person with the view that they have become unreachable. As the work of Richards and Tomandl (2006) signifies it is possible to reach out and establish a connection, even in the later stages of dementia. It requires the will to keep trying and to not give up as difficulties mount, and we can learn a lot from the maintained communicative approaches which are being used by some to connect with individuals in a coma (Mindell 1997). The value here for the person with dementia is that no matter how impaired their cognition they can potentially gain comfort from the attempts by others to reach out and form a connection with them within their increasing isolation.

One approach of much value where communication has become impaired is that of validation, which focuses primarily upon a feelings-based connection. The importance of this is expressed by Bowlby (1988: 156) in that:

> There are, in fact no more important communications between one human being and another than those expressed emotionally, and no information more vital for constructing and reconstructing working models of self and other than information about how each feels toward the other.

The use of validation in later stages of dementia or, as Feil (1993) states, with those who have developed a vegetative state, has the goal of trying to elicit some facial movement – i.e. through smiling, crying or singing – or physical movement in hands and feet. The approach is to centre all of one's energy on the other person by using techniques such as touch or music for brief, focused periods of time. We can also consider other techniques such as multi-sensory stimulation. The essence is that we as carers should endeavour to maintain connection no matter how impaired or unresponsive the individual appears to be. It is when we stop looking for the *person* within the condition that the very humanness of that person begins to disappear.

Attraction

An issue that has partially been addressed previously and one that significantly influences the process of engagement relates to the degree of attractiveness that another person presents to us. The concept of attraction can be looked at through many different facets and is not related solely to a person's appearance or behaviour. It relates essentially to how the other person makes us feel and aspects such as whether or not we seek out their company above and beyond our scheduled care activities with them. It is perhaps true to say that among the various individuals with dementia that we work with there will be some that we prefer spending time with and some that we don't. The reasons for this may be many, and different for each member of the care team.

Activity 7.9

➡ Think about some of the individuals experiencing dementia that you have worked with and consider what determines their sense of attractiveness to you.

I prefer working with some individuals because ...

➡ ....
➡ ....
➡ ....
➡ ....

I find it less appealing or difficult to work with others because ...

➡ ....
➡ ....
➡ ....
➡ ....

With regards to the *prefer working with* list you might have indicated factors such as having a clearly defined role and actually being able to help those you feel nurturing towards. A core aspect here relates to the carer feeling purposeful, valued and needed. We can suppose that within each therapeutic encounter there is to a certain degree a 'what's in it for me' component. It is when the balance between what we *give* and what we *receive* tips dramatically away from the latter that we begin to struggle. No matter how caring or altruistic our intentions, we still need to achieve a sense of purposeful result from the process of caring. It is obviously dependent upon a variety of individual factors and dynamics such as Malan's (2004) *helping profession syndrome*, a process whereby professionals seek to give to others in part the care that they would like to have for themselves. As this in many cases leads to a deficit in the emotional balance of payments, what is important here is the sense of satisfaction or personal gratification that carers are able to get from feeling that others are being helped and that one has actually made a difference. In a number of cases this might relate to working with individuals who are less impaired and able to participate in developing an effective working relationship. These factors help to make the carer feel good about the person worked with and subsequently stimulate a more motivated approach to care.

On the other hand, when considering *those I find less appealing or difficult to work with*, you might have listed such factors as individuals who are significantly impaired and heavily dependent upon others for most aspects of care. Deficits with communication and understanding are especially difficult to deal with as are caring for those who are for example aggressive or sexually disinhibited. For some carers, the person with dementia who is doubly incontinent, unable to converse verbally and has to be assisted with most physical activities of daily living will pose an unattractive proposition. This is because of the heavy demands placed upon a person's already overloaded time as well as the patient's inability to give much that is tangible back. We can relate this to Pavlov's (1958) process of classical conditioning with the reinforcement of the association between *person with dementia* and *unpleasant and demanding tasks*. It does all have an effect on the carer who sees subsequent contact with a specific patient as an unpleasant or unwelcome experience. This is very different than for example the care provided to others who are easier and more gratifying to care for.

Another challenging area for carers emerges when those with dementia 'resist' being looked after. The reasons behind their response might of course be due to many understandable factors such as a fear of losing independence, especially if it is something that has been important for them throughout their life. In many cases though, the gradual deterioration of function and intellect with dementia makes care demoralizing, especially with the assumption that care demands will continue to increase. The highly dependent individual places exhausting demands upon carers and it can be hard to retain a sense of the *person* residing within the condition of *dementia*. This is also compounded by the consequences of a person's condition with aspects such as feeding apraxia where the person has a reduced ability to chew and swallow food and thereby loses skills for feeding themselves in a socially accepted way (Wilbourn and Prosser 2003).

It is worth at this point reflecting upon Felicity Stockwell's (1984) list of factors categorized as representing popular and unpopular patients (see Box 7.1).

Box 7.1 Popular and unpopular patients (Stockwell 1984)

Popular (themes)

- Converse freely
- Know the nurse's name
- Able to joke and laugh with the nurses
- Cooperate in being helped to get well and express determination to do so
- Reward nurses

Unpopular (themes)

- Foreign patients
- In hospital for more than three months
- Patients with a psychiatric diagnosis
- Patients who had attempted suicide

(Behaviours included being grumpy, complaining about the ward/treatment or demanding attention)

If we glance at this list we can certainly assume that for many carers, people experiencing dementia will vary from one category to the other but as the condition deteriorates they are likely to gravitate towards the *unpopular*. There are a number of issues being reflected here such as Talcott Parsons' (1951) notion of the *sick role*, with the implied obligation of playing a part in improving one's condition. Other expectations might centre around the person with dementia showing compliance, being amenable and non-complaining, offering thanks and gratitude or simply allowing carers to help. There is an element here of the person having a role with regards to what they are expected to give back to the carer in order to maintain the sought-after balance in this relationship. It does not account for a multitude of factors whereby the individual is unwilling or simply unable to comply with these demands. For example, the most obvious factor is the level of a person's cognitive deterioration and their confusion or misperception regarding the cues around them. Even well-meaning interventions can be perceived as intimidating and consequently pushed away.

Within the overall theme of attraction is the notion concerning the degree to which we actually like the other person we are working with. This in a number of cases extends beyond their actual appearance and presentation and includes previous factors such as lifestyle, sexuality and occupation among others.

Conclusion

This chapter has focused upon the process of engagement which involves the development of a connection with those experiencing dementia. What is vital here is that this connection is felt and appreciated by others, otherwise their growing sense and feeling of isolation is not going to be impacted upon. Healthcare professionals should be cognizant of some of the potential difficulties which might be located within their own approach, the health state of the person with dementia or the environment within which care is delivered. Engaging with the person and helping them to feel properly supported incorporates using approaches such as empathy and validation, although attention is needed as to what these terms actually mean and how to apply them appropriately in practice.

Key points

- The term 'personality clash' might be applied to relationships too quickly. Instead we should strive to look at and tackle the factors that might be making the process dissatisfying for both those with dementia and ourselves.
- We need to be mindful of how our attempts at engagement might sometimes be misperceived by those we are trying to support. This means being adaptable and also being able to withstand rejection on the patient's part.
- We can engage to varying degrees with *all* people with dementia no matter what their level of confusion. We just need to be more patient and creative in our approach.

References

Bowlby, J. (1988) *A Secure Base: Clinical Applications of Attachment Theory*. London: Routledge.

Cassedy, P. and Cutliffe, J. (1998) Empathy, students and the problems of genuineness, *Mental Health Practice*, 1(9): 28–33.

Davis, R. (1989) *My Journey into Alzheimer's Disease*. Bucks: Tyndale House.

DoH (Department of Health) (2001) *National Service Framework for Older People*. London: DoH.

DoH (Department of Health) (2006) *Participation in Action on Mental Health – A Guide to Promoting Social Inclusion*, www.socialexclusion.gov.uk/downloaddoc.asp?id=300, accessed 28 April 2006.

DoH (Department of Health) (2009) *National Dementia Strategy*. London: DoH.

Feil, N. (1993) *The Validation Breakthrough: Simple Techniques for Communicating with People with 'Alzheimer's-Type Dementia'*. London: Health Professions Press.

Gladstein, G. (1983) Understanding empathy: integrating counseling, developmental, and social psychology perspectives, *Journal of Counseling Psychology*, 30(4): 467–82.

Goldsmith, M. (1996) *Hearing the Voice of People with Dementia: Opportunities and Obstacles*. London: Jessica Kingsley.

Goffman, E. (1961) *Asylums*. Harmondsworth: Penguin.

Hamdy, R. (1998) Clinical presentation, in R. Hamdy, J. Turnbull, J. Edwards and M. Lancaster (eds) *Alzheimer's Disease: A Handbook for Carers*, 3rd edn. London: Mosby.

Jacques, A. (1992) *Understanding Dementia*. Edinburgh: Churchill Livingstone.

Killick, J. and Allan, K. (2001) *Communication and the Care of People with Dementia*. Buckingham: Open University Press.

King, D. and Wertheimer, M. (2005) *Max Wertheimer and Gestalt Theory*. London: Transaction Publishers.

Kitwood, T. (1997) *Dementia Reconsidered*. Buckingham: Open University Press.

Lawton, M.P. and Nahemow, L. (1973) Ecology and the aging process, in C. Eisdorder and M.P. Lawton (eds) *Psychology of Adult Development and Aging*. Washington, DC: American Psychological Association.

Luft, J. and Ingram, H. (1955) *The Johari Window: A Graphic Model for Interpersonal Relations*. Berkeley, CA: University of California, Western Training Lab.

Malan, D. (2004) *Individual Psychotherapy and the Science of Psychodynamics*, 3rd edn. London: Butterworth Heinemann.

Maslow, A. (1970) *Motivation and Personality*, 2nd edn. London: Harper & Row.

Mindell, A. (1997) *Coma, a Healing Journey: A Guide for Families, Friends and Carers*. Portland, OR: Lao Tse Press.

Moos, R. and Lemke, S. (1985) Specialised living environments for older people, in J. Birren and K. Schaie (eds) *Handbook of the Psychology of Ageing.* New York: Reinhold.

O'Connor, J. and Seymour, J. (1990) *Introducing Neurolinguistic Programming. Psychological Skills for Understanding and Influencing People.* London: Aquarian.

Parsons, T. (1951) *The Social System.* Glencoe, IL: Free Press.

Pavlov, I. (1958) *Experimental Psychology and Other Essays.* London: Peter Owen.

Perrin, T. (1997) Occupational need in severe dementia, *Journal of Advanced Nursing,* 25: 934–41.

Phair, L. and Good, V. (1995) *Dementia: A Positive Approach.* London: Scutari Press.

Richards, T. and Tomandl, S. (2006) *An Alzheimer's Surprise Party,* www.tomrichards.com/publications.htm, accessed 1 February 2009.

Rogers, C. (1961) *On Becoming a Person: A Therapist's View of Psychotherapy.* Boston, MA: Houghton Mifflin.

Stockwell, F. (1984) *The Unpopular Patient.* London: Croom Helm.

Truax, C. (1961) A scale for the measurement of accurate empathy, *Psychiatric Institute Bulletin,* 1: 12.

Wilbourn, M. and Prosser, S. (2003) *The Pathology and Pharmacology of Mental Illness.* Cheltenham: Nelson Thornes.

Zimmerman, S., Williams, C., Reed, P., Boustani, M., Preisser, J., Heck, E. and Sloane, P. (2005) Attitudes, stress and satisfaction of staff who care for residents with dementia, *The Gerontologist,* 45: 96–105.

Further reading

Gillies, C. and James, A. (1994) *Reminiscence Work with Old People.* London: Chapman & Hall.

8 Empowerment and disempowerment

Objectives: After reading this chapter you should be able to:

- Discuss what types of interventions and approaches can be used to help empower those with dementia.
- Explore how the assessment of a person's vulnerabilities and risk factors can influence professional judgements and paternalistic responses.
- Reflect upon what the notion of empowerment means to the person who has a diagnosis of dementia.

A clinical dilemma (practitioner's perspective)

'I want to maintain Arthur's autonomy although I am mindful about how vulnerable he is because of his deteriorating cognitive state.'

'My concerns are heightened where those I am caring for are experiencing recent or long-term mental health problems and physical frailties.'

'Determining the extent of what those with dementia can safely do is problematic and might be influenced by the ways in which we seek to understand the impact that their cognitive problems have upon them.'

'Safeguarding the "best interests" of the person with dementia and acknowledging my "duty of care" is stressed by various professional and political structures and should therefore take precedence.'

And yet ... we should not forget the impact that 'risk management' approaches have on the person with dementia and should carefully weigh them up against the resultant loss of freedom and autonomy.

Introduction

This chapter builds upon a variety of themes which have been previously covered such as the range of attitudes held about people with dementia and an appreciation of their felt and lived experience. Related activities and exercises have provided ways of engaging with those experiencing cognitive and communication deficits and have highlighted the need to seek and develop an understanding of the person and their views on their world. It is a process which is enabled through the development of an effective therapeutic relationship between healthcare staff and those with dementia. What is important within this relationship is the degree of autonomy or control held by each party. It is often the case that people with dementia feel undermined or disempowered as others take over, because of the generally low expectations and negative assumptions commonly held about those with this condition. The term dementia is equated here with concepts such as helplessness or 'at risk' and leads towards disempowering and dependency-fostering approaches being adopted. Our need as carers is to support the person with dementia in retaining as much control as is possible over their lives. The core issue explored within this chapter is the process of empowerment and the ways in which it is either promoted or obstructed in practice.

Figure 8.1 considers factors that could impact on how empowerment is perceived and maintained following healthcare professionals' judgements and actions. Empowerment and self-determination rights are strongly influenced by assessments about potential risk and the potential levels of vulnerability regarding those concerned. Striving to balance *empowerment* and *vulnerability* concerns can be problematic as we attempt to maintain self-determination rights yet at the same time being mindful of potential difficulties and legislative issues.

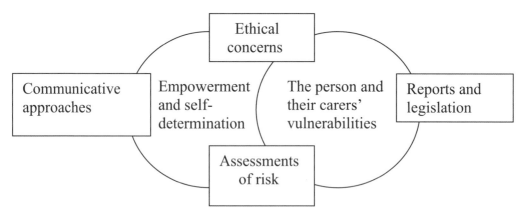

Figure 8.1 Empowerment

Activity 8.1

➡ You may find it helpful to access the internet website Dementia Advocacy and Support Network International at www.dasninternational.org. This is a worldwide organization for people diagnosed with dementia, and those who work within comparable services that advocate on their behalf.

The struggle for empowerment is something which individuals can experience from the moment of diagnosis, when common assumptions about their condition can cause others to relegate their qualities, skills and capabilities behind their deficits, struggles and difficulties. The generally low expectations and concerns that others hold can be transferred to the person with dementia and influence how autonomous they remain. Lubinski (1991) proposed that learned behaviours may arise as a consequence of the perceptions or beliefs adopted by others and that 'learned helplessness' and a cycle of incompetence can be triggered by the diagnosis of dementia. We can regard the process of learned helplessness as occurring when the person with dementia believes that outcomes and events are not being determined by their own actions. This in turn generates feelings of being unable to determine present and future intentions and the planning and implementation of further actions seems futile. The daily interactions and decision-making choices the person with dementia undertakes may well influence how they engage with others, either maintaining an independent stance or developing permission-seeking behaviours which promote dependence on other people. In a study of 17 people with the early diagnosis of Alzheimer's disease it was found that disempowerment, labelling, stigmatization and feelings of banishment characterized social interactions. These expressions resulted in insults to the person's self-identity and sense of control (Harris and Sterin 1999).

Embracing notions of empowerment

In order to embrace notions of empowerment there is a requirement to seek ways of developing caring partnerships which challenge (or at least question) the power variables that exist between a person with dementia and healthcare professionals. You might have particular feelings and thoughts about the degree of control and the extent to which we can embrace a more person-centred partnership. Giving the person with dementia and their family carers greater control over their lives is an important aspect in maintaining well-being and independence. Recognizing that the person with dementia retains rights to make decisions and choices incorporates an awareness of established, new and even predicted limitations that their health state might foster. Notwithstanding the impact dementia can have, we seek to engage with and promote opportunities for autonomous decision-making while also safeguarding a person's health and well-being. Embracing an empowering approach also challenges a number of long-established ageist attitudes which are held towards older people within society.

Activity 8.2

From the following words, which do you feel underpin empowering actions and why?

➡ Allowing
➡ Delegating
➡ Enabling

> ➡ Permitting
> ➡ Authorizing
> ➡ Entitling
> ➡ Qualifying

The term 'empowerment' has numerous meanings but two distinct features:

1 *The having and sharing of power* – this includes the degree of control a person with dementia might hold over a range of decisions including treatment options.
2 *Sources of power and ways of increasing that power* – this includes education/information-giving, for example about a person's legal rights.

A further view could be to consider empowerment as a social process of recognizing, promoting and enhancing a person's ability to meet their needs, solve their problems and mobilize the necessary resources in order to feel in control of their lives (Gibson 1991). This sees the process of empowerment as involving an external party who enables and supports a person to take control of their own life.

Exercise 1: Debating empowerment

This exercise details a debating forum which was set up to explore healthcare students' understanding of the term empowerment and the potential benefits for the person with dementia and their carers (full details are provided in Chapter 9). Two groups were encouraged to consider opposing points of view and rationales:

• *Position A: why is empowerment important for the person with dementia?* This position is concerned with reinforcing self-determination rights, maintaining the person's decision-making capabilities and keeping the working relationships on an equal status.
• *Position B: why is it less risky and easier to do things for the person with dementia?* This position is concerned with a person's cognitive decline and subsequent 'risky' behaviours. Professional issues of accountability and responsibility (duty of care) are highlighted here.

This exercise promoted a lively debate between students' representations of these two competing viewpoints. The group supporting position A outlined the limited power held by those with dementia and their struggle to gain a sense of control. They argued fairly passionately on behalf of those who should be allowed greater freedom and choice about their care but who tend to be dismissed and ignored because of stereotypical notions about their fading capabilities. The other group representing position B were very much concerned with the question of professional accountability, fearing critical responses from relatives or potential lawsuits should any harm befall individuals in their care. The attitude 'we know best' seemed to be encouraged here because of the greater measure of security and control provided for those giving care. The debate and reflection around this exercise prompted students to become more mindful of the dilemma facing those providing care as well as increasing their awareness about the experience of those with dementia.

The balance of power between the healthcare professional and the person with dementia can be a delicate one, with the experience of dementia playing a part in hindering and obstructing self-empowerment. Goldsmith (1996) argued that people with dementia are often disempowered in two ways, firstly by their illness and secondly by other people's reactions. As an individual practitioner you may have worked in healthcare teams that uphold traditional paternalistic care approaches where decisions are made on behalf of those with dementia because the healthcare professional 'knows best'. In such circumstances this unshifting position of dominance may well promote disempowerment. Altering the balance is a complex process and individual practitioners or healthcare teams can exercise power consciously or unconsciously; it can be overt and openly displayed, latent and subconscious, but nonetheless pervasive (Canter 2001; Palvianen et al. 2003). Furthermore, personal and behavioural complexities allied to how the person with dementia experiences their world and the people within it can add a further clinical dynamic where risk and vulnerability influence the degree of self-determination and independence promoted. Pearlin et al. (2001) argued that there was a tendency for generalizations to be of a bleak prognosis with assumptions that all people with dementia are unable to express their needs and are seen as passive objects on whose behalf decisions should be made and actions taken.

Empowerment approaches and ethical actions

The word autonomy is often broadly defined as: 'self determination, self rule, being your own person' (Parker and Dickenson 2001: 136). Society places a high worth on autonomous beliefs where citizens are able to make choices about their own lifestyles. Autonomy literally means 'self-rule', derived from the Greek words *autos* (self) and *nomo* (rule, governance or law). Within these principles of autonomy there is an implication that people have the freedom to decide how they manage their lives and as Farsides (2002: 123) relates: 'to be autonomous is to fit into the picture of what it means to be an effective and successful member of society'. From a healthcare perspective the principles of respect for autonomy can be demonstrated by treating a person with dementia as somebody with rights and not simply as an object of care. This stance embraces a person-centred philosophy of care which has specific central beliefs that acknowledge an individual's rights to hold their own views, make choices and take actions based upon their personal values and beliefs. Respect for a person's autonomy and their right to consent to or refuse treatment are central tenets in healthcare, with guidelines recommending a greater service-user involvement within the decision-making process (HPC 2002; NMC 2008). This enhances the view of an autonomous person as someone who lives their life according to their own values and aspirations.

The scope of paternalism varies and a consensus view suggests that these interventions involve acting against another's choices for their own benefit or to prevent harm to them. Beauchamp and Childress (2001: 178) offer the following definition: 'The intentional overriding of one person's preferences or actions by another person. Where the person who overrides this justifies the action by the goal of benefiting or avoiding harm to the person whose preferences or actions are overridden'. From a healthcare perspective, interventions of this kind should be formulated from an objective view of what would be of best interest for the person being cared for, based upon discovering their wants and needs and those of their carers.

Figure 8.2. considers a variety of ethical actions that healthcare professionals could explore. The four outer boxes provide explanations of various approaches which care staff could take regarding designated community concerns such as:

- evidence of the person wandering around the streets at night-time;
- increased hostility towards neighbours and strangers;
- concerns about the safety of the carer.

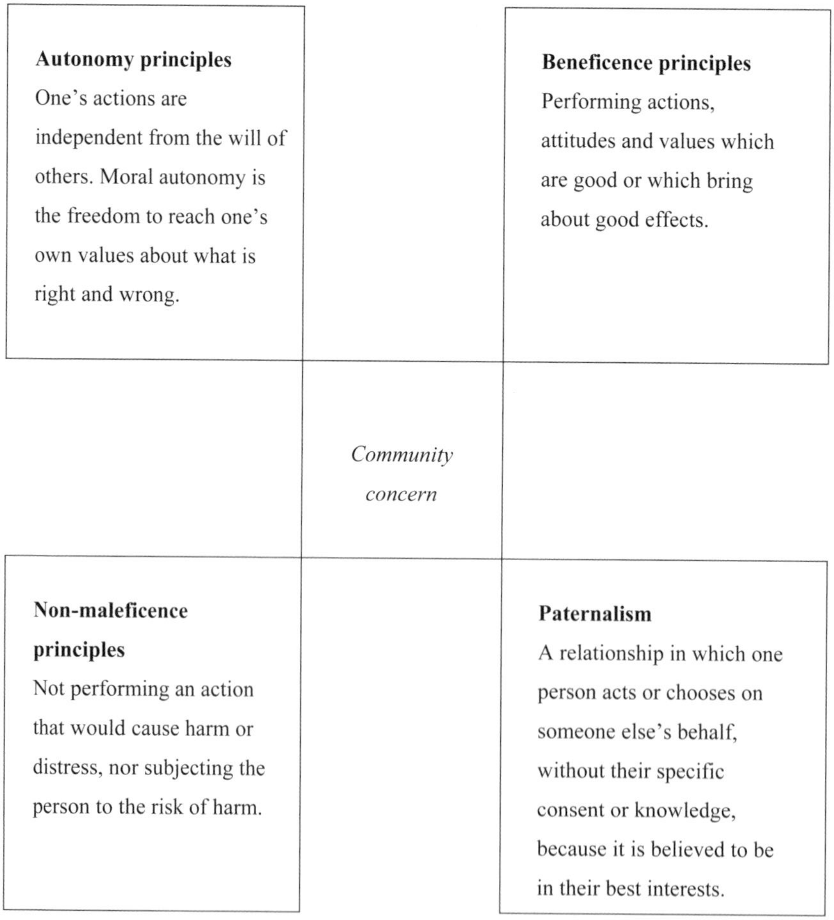

Autonomy principles		Beneficence principles
One's actions are independent from the will of others. Moral autonomy is the freedom to reach one's own values about what is right and wrong.		Performing actions, attitudes and values which are good or which bring about good effects.
	Community concern	
Non-maleficence principles		Paternalism
Not performing an action that would cause harm or distress, nor subjecting the person to the risk of harm.		A relationship in which one person acts or chooses on someone else's behalf, without their specific consent or knowledge, because it is believed to be in their best interests.

Figure 8.2 Community concerns

When considering various *community concerns* it is important to be cognizant of the difficulties in balancing often opposing views and facts. As soon as a person's autonomy is impaired their involvement in decision-making processes can become reduced. This can also impact upon and limit the choices they make with the potential for their requests to become overruled or discounted. A moral justification for acting without the consent from the person with dementia can be argued where principles of a duty to do no harm (non-maleficence) and a duty to do good (beneficence) exist. Bond *et al.* (2002) argued that in everyday life the labelling of someone as having dementia and the taken-for-granted assumption that they will lack insight has profound implications for their independence and autonomy.

Activity 8.3

Arthur is occasionally becoming forgetful, losing personal items (including house keys) and once forgot to switch off the gas cooker.

Can you justify a need for paternalism?

➡ I can because …
➡ I cannot because …
➡ I am unsure because …

As highlighted by Activity 8.3, concerns about a person's safety might cause family or professional caregivers to conclude that beneficence or non-maleficence outweigh the person's autonomy. These thoughts are often construed in terms of levels of risk, which cross a threshold for the caregiver of unacceptable danger (Woods and Pratt 2005). See Best Fit 8.1 for practice recommendations.

Best Fit 8.1

There are no simple solutions to the complexities of Arthur's present health status and the potential risks as a consequence of his forgetfulness. You may have considered the following conditions:

• Is Arthur at risk of significant and preventable harm?
• Will the types of paternalistic interventions employed have a probability of preventing harm?
• Has Arthur the capacity for rational reflection or are his cognitive abilities impaired?
• Do the benefits to Arthur of these types of interventions outweigh his present forgetfulness and risks?

In Chapter 4 we visited Elsie at a point prior to her admission into residential care. The information in Case Study 8.1 provides additional details written by the healthcare student visiting her at home.

Case Study 8.1

To recap: Elsie is an 83-year-old widower experiencing dementia. Prior to her admission she had been visited at home by a healthcare student and community psychiatric nurse who were alarmed at the untidy and chaotic state of her house (including litter and rotting food).

Elsie

Even though I reminded Elsie of the unhealthy way she was living, she said she was not bothered by these conditions. She was financially astute and was able to manage her affairs competently. Furthermore, she was adamant that her house was perfectly liveable and took exception to being told it was in need of attention. Consequently, she took no responsibility for the condition of her house, did not believe there was a health risk, and refused to allow the council entry into her property in order to clean it.

Elsie was reminded that there would not be a charge for the work to be undertaken by the council workers; at hearing this she became visibly distressed, stating she did not require charity and didn't want strangers entering her house. At this point she asked me to leave.

Activity 8.2 asked you to think about actions that could enhance empowering interventions. You may well have concluded that most if not all of these words were pertinent. With this in mind, having now been provided with further information about Elsie's lifestyle, consider the questions in Activity 8.4.

Activity 8.4

Have your views towards Elsie changed?

➡ Should she be allowed to continue her lifestyle with minimal interference (yet continued support) from healthcare professionals?
➡ Should healthcare professionals take stronger and more urgent actions?

Professional and ethical tensions may surface when striving to find a balance between Elsie's autonomy and the greater public good, especially where judgements and attitudes focus on the degree of risk and potential harm her actions could cause to herself and others: 'The drive to avoid harm provides a push towards removal of autonomy, and to generalise from the loss of some competences to other or all areas of function' (Woods and Pratt 2005: 428). When there is reluctance from individuals with mental health problems to engage with service providers a number of difficulties are posed because of the ethical and legal issues involved in the assessment of risk (Gunstone 2003). An act of paternalism, which necessitates the exercise of professional power and authority, may be justified if the person is experiencing certain degrees of mental health problems which diminish their capacity to act in an autonomous manner (Fulford 1995). Furthermore, the psychological experiences of specific psychiatric symptoms (hallucinations, delusions and depression) can reduce a person's capacity to govern themselves and act in an autonomous manner (Beauchamp 2000). See Best Fit 8.2 for practice recommendations.

Best Fit 8.2

There are no simple solutions to the complexities of Elsie's present health status and living conditions. Here are some suggestions.

- Maintaining Elsie in her house would not cause the distress of being rehoused or temporarily placed in health/social care and this could retain her independent lifestyle.
- Encouraging Elsie to seek assistance with the condition of the house and regular support in maintaining a more healthy environment.
- Frequent monitoring of Elsie's mental health state and the cognitive implications of the recent diagnosis of early-onset dementia.
- Listen, advise and offer Elsie a strategy/management plan for continuing her independence while also retaining relationships.

The nature of risk

If you pick up a newspaper, listen to the radio, watch the television or access the internet on the reporting of local and national events you are provided with a daily reminder that we live in risky times. We are often presented with images and messages that create an alarmist view, less about reassurance and more about the describing of human frailties and calamitous events. The plight of older people living in the community is often represented as a group who are vulnerable and therefore susceptible to the risks of daily living. An earlier view provides an uncomfortable image of frailty and vulnerability shown towards older people: 'Responses to these images express either paternalistic concerns with protection, or equally paternalistic promotion of risk-taking. Both positions fail to take into account the ability of older people to make their own decisions' (Reed 1998: 251).

World concerns relating to pollution, populations and political propagandas may occupy our thoughts and concerns as much as smoking-related diseases, childhood obesity, the increase in diagnoses of dementia (with incidences seeming to occur earlier in people's lives) and the steadily ageing population. Determining what constitutes risk, and therefore what are risky behaviours, is not always straightforward as they may be perceived differently by different people. Exercise 2 addresses the notion of risk as understood by healthcare students.

Exercise 2: What makes risky behaviours?

This exercise (see Chapter 9 for full details) commenced with healthcare students being asked to write a brief list of the 'risky type' behaviours that they had engaged in over the previous few months. Comments were then shared in pairs and each partner in turn was asked to rate their colleague's behaviours. The range of possible scores was 0–3, 4–7 or 8–10, signifying the possible degrees of risk. These numerical ranges are subjective and suggest low, medium or high concerns. Group feedback and the itemizing of 'What makes risky behaviours?' were presented in a lively fashion with some humour and insightful comments being made during self-disclosure. Risky behaviours included the following: walking alone in unlit areas at night, smoking ten cigarettes a day, going potholing, drinking a lot of alcohol, horse-riding and eating junk food.

These behaviours are not necessarily restricted to particular generations or person-ality types but all carry a potential risk tariff. However, this view might be disputed depending upon how one views these activities with statements about moderation or safety precautions challenging the perceived degree of risk attached. It is interesting to consider how our views become more fearful and protective if the person concerned happens to also have a diagnosis of dementia. This is where we question the person's ability to make informed decisions about their personal risk and become inclined towards taking charge.

The Royal Society (1992: 2) considered risk definitions and associated themes in the following ways:

- risk defined in terms of probability 'that a particular adverse event occurs during a stated period of time, or results from a particular challenge';
- risk assessment is used to 'describe the study of decisions subject to uncertain consequences', being divided into risk estimation (outcomes, magnitude and probability) and risk evaluation (significance or value of significant hazards);
- risk management is 'the making of decisions concerning risks and their subsequent implementation, and flows from risk estimation and risk evaluation'.

These definitions consider risk in objective terms, focusing on single adverse events, and do not necessarily take into consideration the complex variables that exist in real life. Risk assessment should really be looking at *balancing harms and benefits*. Clarke (2000) discusses how risk as constructed and defined by health and social care agencies differs from perceptions held by people with dementia and their carers. Professionals emphasize the physical aspects of safety, while maintaining self-identity and interpersonal relationships are more important to people with dementia and their families. Clarke concludes that there should be a sharing of these different perspectives resulting in improved care outcomes. Assumptions about risk often refer to the likelihood of a negative outcome or form of harm occurring, however in each instance these should be carefully weighed up against the positive outcomes which can ensue when greater freedom and autonomy are promoted.

Activity 8.5

➡ When do you feel risk-taking activities could be beneficial?

Pritchard (1997: 81) considers the risks taken by vulnerable people and argues that:

> *we all take risks to achieve something we want and in many situations we experience various emotions while taking the risk – enjoyment, excitement, fear, anxiety. If we achieve what we want, we then experience a great sense of achievement and fulfilment and we may get approval and respect from others.*

It might be useful here to consider your own observations of healthcare professionals' interpretations and assessments of risk and the degree to which individuals subsequently had further limitations imposed on them. Ethical tensions and professional concerns can manifest themselves when seeking to find the right balance between maintaining the individual's autonomy and self-determination rights and imposing professional or legislative controls, for example through 'duty of care' to safeguard that individual, their carers and possibly neighbours. Dowie (1999) argues that risk is an ambiguous concept that has frequently been used to disempower people by creating an illusion of certainty and control by 'risk experts'. The term 'risk' would appear to have numerous judgemental qualities that often focus on harmful outcomes, hazards and dangers to be avoided, although risk-taking activities may provide potential benefits. Central to these possible contradictions are the abilities of the assessor to understand the world of the person being assessed.

Risk assessment can be a complicated and sometimes lengthy procedure that requires a systematic collection and processing of information allied to the application of the best available evidence-based knowledge. It is a process that requires time to conduct and needs to be offered in a sensitive manner which ultimately seeks to improve predictions. Undertaking clinical assessments usually involves a semi-structured interview with the person with dementia, and where applicable carers and significant others in that person's life. This process will include practice observations which depend upon the healthcare professional's knowledge, experience and judgement. Tools measuring the severity of dementia are included in Box 8.1. These include actuarial risk assessment tools which match the individual with populations based on indicators or 'at risk' factors in a structured framework, using instruments based on statistical data. Clinical judgements focus on factors uniquely related to the person and can include how cognitive impairment impacts on their lifestyle, relationships and the context of how they and their carers cope with the condition of dementia.

Box 8.1 Dementia assessment scales

1   The Global Deterioration Scale (GDS) has seven categories that range from no cognitive decline to very mild – mild – moderate – moderately severe – severe and very severe cognitive decline (Reisberg *et al.* 1982).
2   Bristol Activities of Daily Living Scale: a 20-question assessment with a maximum score of 60 that equates to very severe. The scale covers eating – dressing – personal hygiene – toileting – mobility – orientation – communication – domestic tasks (Bucks *et al.* 1996).
3   BEHAVE-AD is designed to assess behavioural symptoms of patients with Alzheimer's disease. There are 26 questions which cover: delusional ideas – hallucinations – disturbed activity – aggressiveness – sleep and mood disturbances – anxiety symptoms (Reisberg *et al.* 1987).

Activity 8.6

➡   What types of risk assessment tools have you witnessed or been involved in?
➡   Why were they of benefit in determining the person's risk and where did professional judgements appear within the decision-making process?
➡   How and where were these assessments undertaken?

The key issues in the use of risk assessment tools are firstly how effective they are at distinguishing those at risk from those who are not and secondly the extent to which they measure up in terms of efficiency and accuracy against professional judgements. Initial judgements provide a type of assessment focusing upon the person's condition and whether it is improving, remaining stable or deteriorating. The information gathered here can help with subsequent judgements and decisions. The way in which judgements are made and their degree of accuracy is important for clinical practice. A study by Lamond *et al.* (1996) attempted to classify types of judgement:

- *casual judgements* (*diagnosis*) – statements expressing a state or condition based on the presence of attributes which are used to explain a problem;
- *descriptive judgements* – statements expressing a state or condition based on the presence of attributes which have been observed directly or obtained from another source;

- *evaluative judgements* – statements expressing a qualitative difference in a state or condition based on the presence of attributes which have been observed directly or obtained from another source;
- *inference judgements* – statements expressing the presence of a state or condition which are not based on any information gathered from or about the patient.

Figure 8.3. considers the possible outcomes of assessing a person's risk and ideally results in being able to offer positive predictions. Errors in prediction have repercussions in terms of professional accountability as well as creating restrictions for the person with dementia.

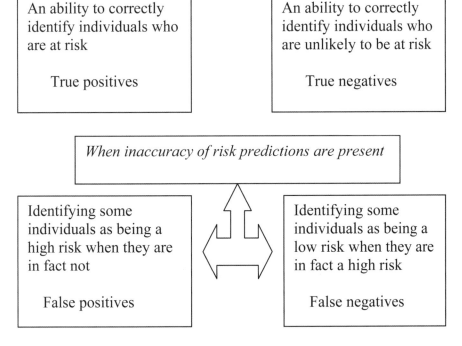

Figure 8.3 Assessing risk

The most comprehensive form of risk assessment combines professional judgement, risk factor identification and the use of risk assessment tools. In simple terms:

the effectiveness of risk assessment tools = ↓ **the number of false positives identified**
+
↓ **the number of false negatives identified**

The ability of assessment tools to identify true positives relates to their degree of accuracy and sensitivity (people who actually have the disease or condition that is being tested for). The ability to identify true negatives relates to specificity (people who do not have the condition or disease that is being tested for).

Activity 8.7

Could there be difficulties (false positives and false negatives) in assessing the risks posed by the behaviours and lifestyles of:

➡ Arthur and his forgetfulness?
➡ Elsie and her lifestyle choices and reluctance to change?

Empowerment through reports and legislation

The need to readdress the imbalance in power between the person with dementia and the healthcare professional is something that has long been recognized within health and social care policies. The 1991 report *Case Management and Assessment: Practitioner's Guide* (DoH 1991) outlines the protagonists as service providers and service users. The shift in the balance of power was given further impetus in *The NHS Plan* (DoH 2000) through increased service user involvement, public participation and advocacy initiatives. Using an autonomous style of language, for example the 'expert patient' and establishing a 'patient-focused NHS', the provision of choice and the promotion of empowerment were attempts at changing the roles of patients.

Activity 8.8

Consider the issues identified in Chapter 10 of *The NHS Plan* (DoH 2000):

➡ information to empower patients;
➡ strengthen patient choice;
➡ protection of patients;
➡ a new patient advocacy service;
➡ rights of redress;
➡ consent;
➡ patients' views;
➡ scrutiny of the NHS;
➡ patient representation throughout the NHS.

Furthermore, the Audit Commission (2002) acknowledged the importance of encouraging empowerment and maximizing the independence and autonomy of people with dementia. The Mental Capacity Act (MCA) 2005, which came into full operation in November 2007, seeks to empower and protect vulnerable people who are not able to make their own decisions. It makes it clear who can take decisions, in which situations, and how they should go about this. It also enables people to plan ahead for a time when they may lose capacity. There are a set of five principles that underpin the MCA:

- a *presumption of capacity* to make decisions unless proved otherwise;
- the right for *individuals to be supported* to make their own decisions before it is concluded that they cannot make decisions for themselves;
- *individuals must retain* the right to make what might be seen to be an eccentric or unwise decision;
- anything that is done for or on behalf of individuals without capacity must be in their *best interests*;
- interventions must be the *least restrictive* alternative in terms of their basic rights and freedoms.

A key area for carers and people with dementia is the issue of decision-making when mental incapacity is questioned.

Activity 8.9

➡ What does decision-making incapacity mean for you?

Guidance on decision-making incapacity states that the person is 'unable by reason of mental disability to make or communicate a decision, where mental disability includes any disability or disorder of mind or brain, permanent or temporary, resulting in an impairment or disturbance of mental functioning' (Lord Chancellor's Department 1999: 8). There may well be potential perceptual difficulties regarding a person's decision-making capacity as illustrated in Ganzini *et al.*'s (2004) study which concluded that clinicians hold certain common myths which influence how subsequent judgements are formed (see Box 8.2).

Box 8.2 Ten myths about decision-making capacity (Ganzini et *al.* 2004)

1 Decision-making capacity and competency are the same.
2 Lack of decision-making capacity can be presumed when patients go against medical advice.
3 There is no need to assess decision-making capacity unless patients go against medical advice.
4 Decision-making capacity is an 'all or nothing' phenomenon.
5 Cognitive impairment equals lack of decision-making capacity.
6 Lack of decision-making capacity is a permanent condition.
7 Patients who have not been given relevant and consistent information about their treatment lack decision-making capacity.
8 All patients with certain psychiatric disorders lack decision-making capacity.

9   Patients who are involuntarily committed lack decision-making capacity.
10 Only mental health experts can assess decision-making capacity.

The MCA also includes the legal authority for carers to make day-to-day decisions on behalf of someone who lacks capacity and who has nominated someone to make decisions on their behalf. From April 2007 health and social care professionals have been required to follow a code of practice. Government intentions in August 2007 were to develop the first National Dementia Strategy and an implementation plan for England. In February 2009, *Living Well with Dementia: A New Dementia Strategy* (DoH 2009) was published and seeks to significantly improve dementia care services across three key areas:

- improved awareness and understanding;
- earlier diagnosis and intervention;
- a higher quality of care.

Activity 8.10

Have a look at the following two documents online:

➡ The MCA is available from www.dca.gov.uk/menincap/bill-summary.htm.
➡ Information on the Dementia Strategy is available from
   www.dh.gov.uk/en/Publicationsandstatistics/Publications/
   Public.ationsPolicyAndGuidance/DH_094058.

Communication and empowerment

In order for empowering approaches to be properly promoted in practice it is essential that we facilitate communication with the person experiencing dementia. Empowerment entails a sharing of power with those we are working with and therefore requires there to be a clear flow of understanding between both parties involved. While the cognitive deficiencies associated with dementia can promote certain communication difficulties, problems can also be located within the healthcare professional's approach – i.e. pattern of speech and type of language used. Communication is a dynamic process forever changing as we adjust or adapt our language to the circumstances or situations we find ourselves in. The ways in which we communicate can be influenced by such unique factors as our own life history, past experiences and events as well as the social roles that have formed part of our existence. Each generation has its own cultural values and beliefs that influence the ways they view or develop stereotypical attitudes towards a person or group of people. These opinions about stereotypical social roles can have an influence on the ways we communicate and respond to each other.

Where language barriers exist, advice and guidance concerning treatment may not be fully understood with psychological support being limited and privacy and confidentiality compromised (Gerrish 2001).

Activity 8.11

What might be the consequences for the person with dementia if you were to use the following language approaches:

➡ an over-reliance on medical and/or technical jargon;
➡ providing detailed information such as signs, symptoms, medication;
➡ conversations conducted in a quick manner;
➡ an over-familiarity of address.

Activity 8.11 asks you to consider some of the consequences for the person with dementia when faced with particular language approaches. To look at what the impact here is you might want to consider times in your life when you met a person who held a more senior professional status to yourself (e.g. teacher to student, doctor to patient) who talked at you in a style that was somewhat patronizing or demeaning with an over-use of language you were unaccustomed to. Your feelings would probably fit one of the following:

• comfortable with yourself and the other person;
• an equal partner in the conversation;
• intimidated and unable to express your thoughts and feelings.

It is the third option here which is currently characterized by the type of interaction the person with dementia encounters with healthcare professionals. This section can be summed up by: 'In any relationship, language can be used to exert control over another individual, not necessarily with any malicious intent – it may simply be an anxiety containment function when there is uncertainty about how to react to a given situation' (Miller 2002: 49). Recommendations for practice are provided in Best Fit 8.3.

Best Fit 8.3

• Consider where conversations take place and the presence of distractions, interruptions and background noises.
• Ensure that your language is adaptable enough to accommodate the other person's understanding, acknowledging sensory and speech difficulties, cognitive impairments and where the person's first language is not English.
• Check the other person's comprehension of what is being discussed.
• Regulate the pace of the conversion so as to minimize frustrating, confusing or exhausting the other person.

- Seek permission from the person as to their preferred form of address. Not all people who have cause to access health services are welcoming of over-familiarity.

It is not always a given that a person who has contact with healthcare professionals is unable to properly communicate. However, factors such as status or roles can influence how expressed messages are interpreted by both parties. There is a potential for social isolation if a person loses their abilities to speak and be understood. As Wise (2003: 95) highlights: 'the human dependence on the spoken word explains why deafness isolates more than blindness'. The intensity of our verbal and non-verbal interactions allow us to tell the person with dementia that they remain valued. Sabat and Harré (1992) argue that people with dementia, like everyone else, rely on social exchanges with others to establish and maintain a sense of identity, but are less likely to meet with cooperative responses necessary for the construction of a valid identity. Listening has a crucial role to play in the communication process as feeling acknowledged by others can encourage us to talk. As well as assisting us with expressing our feelings we can also feel respected and valued. If we sense that we are not being listened to then initially feelings may gravitate around the other person not being interested in us as a person, or what we have to say. There is a difference between listening and hearing and as Eckes (1996) suggests, hearing takes place through the operation of a sensory apparatus which allows sound waves to enter the brain. Listening, however, is an *active skill* – it is an art which can be developed through practice, in that it can become a stance, a position or an attitude that we can choose to take or not and in order to listen we must really want to do so (Gordon 1999). Figure 8.4 considers the human complexities surrounding the ways good listening behaviours are developed.

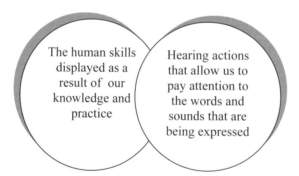

The human skills displayed as a result of our knowledge and practice

Hearing actions that allow us to pay attention to the words and sounds that are being expressed

Figure 8.4 Listening behaviours

Good listening skills convey important messages and by showing full attention the healthcare professional is stating a genuine interest in the other person and a willingness to try and see the world from their perspective. The use of body language behaviours (e.g. nodding, mirrored movements, eye contact and a close proximity) can serve as observable prompts that encourage acknowledgement of the other person while also reinforcing that you are attending to their views and mannerisms by not exhibiting distracting behaviours (e.g. fidgeting, looking disinterested, forgetting what has been said). The degree to which a person is able to communicate their thoughts and feelings may well determine how much they can be 'heard' by others. Communication is an area in which practitioners often fail to meet the person with dementia's needs and poor communication between healthcare professionals and service-users/carers is a frequent cause of complaints (Health Service Ombudsman for England 2003). Communication with a person and their dementia is essential as any impairment may limit a person's ability and willingness to express themselves and prove damaging to their confidence and self-esteem (Miller 2002). Listening and being willing to understand the person's perceptions and lived experiences assists in interpreting their behaviours and interpretations of their world.

The ability to communicate with people who have dementia needs to be continuously developed through education, training and clinical supervision. This process may well begin with a belief that we can become effective communicators even though we may have to accommodate the other person's sensory impairment, confusion and other communicative deficits.

Activity 8.12

Communication can be regarded as having three distinct elements:

➡ *Verbal* – allows words, phrases, colloquialisms to be used.
➡ *Visual* – includes body movements, posture, gestures, touch, and facial expressions.
➡ *Vocal* – determines the voice pitch, speed, volume and tone.

Look at each of these three communicative elements in turn and consider:

➡ How they can have empowering qualities.
➡ How they can have disempowering qualities.

Activity 8.12 considers the different modes of speech comprising verbal, visual and vocal components. The way that we use these has an impact upon the overall message received by the other person. Adapting our speech patterns towards another person can exert different influences that may prove beneficial or detrimental in the long term. Speech accommodation theory was described by Thakerar *et al.* (1982) and proposed that people modify aspects of their speech so that it conforms more to the way their conversational partner speaks, possibly as a way of achieving social approval. This could create a wide range of subtle adaptations that tend to occur more or less unconsciously, although when people meet for the first time these evaluations can potentially be based on stereotypes. This is known as *convergence* and is not necessarily an automatic feature of all conversations, and can be influenced by the social context people find themselves in. A different form of speech diversity is *divergence* where the speaker accentuates their verbal and non-verbal differences in order to distinguish themselves from others. A person's pattern of speech therefore may provide clues about their evaluation of another person's competence and status. Figure 8.5 identifies how the accommodation process can occur.

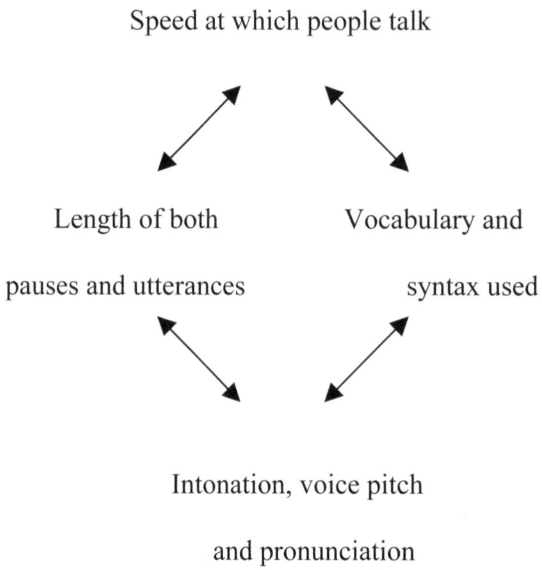

Speed at which people talk

Length of both

pauses and utterances

Vocabulary and

syntax used

Intonation, voice pitch

and pronunciation

Figure 8.5 Accommodation process

From a practitioner's perspective, the use of over-accommodation speech can be a disempowering approach that employs subtle and effective techniques for exercising influence and control. Within speech accommodation theory, the term over-accommodation refers to a particular pattern of speech modification that sometimes characterizes how older people are addressed (Edwards and Noller 1998). Elements of this approach could include the use of simplified vocabulary accompanied by relatively slow speech and possibly placing an exaggerated stress on certain words. An increased use of repetition and adopting an authoritative manner could underpin these interactions. In addition, there may be a tendency to place exaggerated stress on certain words, and an increased use of imperatives, questions and repetition (Edwards and Noller 1998). The adoption of this speech style may be partly grounded within an ethos of controlling patterns of care, where the functional purposes of the institution (agenda of the service) and the attitudes of individual practitioners (personal agendas) underpin the types of interventions used. Older people's services have in the past suffered from this language approach and this may have contributed to the quality of care provided. The use of this type of language could engender dependence upon the practitioner while also lowering the person's self-esteem. One of the key findings from the report *Living Well into Later Life* highlights that despite the changes that have been implemented across healthcare ageism remains within all services and this translates to patronizing and thoughtless treatment from staff (Commission for Healthcare Audit and Inspection 2006).

Conclusion

The experience of dementia along with its associated losses of function, ability and role is in itself an extremely disempowering process. It is vital therefore when contemplating the support of those with dementia to look at ways to promote independence, provide choices and options and help to maintain personal integrity. The acts or conditions that promote empowerment can be important for the well-being of the person with dementia, but need to be implemented in a sensitive manner so as not to engender feelings of helplessness. This process can entail a delicate balance of promoting freedom and autonomy while at the same time being mindful of the person's vulnerabilities and potential risk factors. Assessing the risks to the person with dementia can involve a complex series of activities which weigh up the person's wants, fears and doubts against a decline in their cognitive abilities, possible physical frailties and a shift towards dependence upon health and social care services. Arguably similar themes of wants, fears and doubts in determining what could serve the person's 'best interests' may be influenced by the assessor's use of risk assessment tools and the professional judgements made. When interpreting a person's performance and scores from cognitive assessments and testing the following should be taken into account:

- physical or neurological problems;
- past or current mental health problems;
- educational level and language abilities;
- skills, prior level of functioning and attainment.

The assessor's skills are focused upon making judgements in terms of balancing harms and benefits. The 'duty of care' responsibilities that healthcare professionals work with emphasize the need to take risk seriously. If individuals with dementia are to feel fully involved, properly appreciated and acknowledged for what they can do there needs to be a more considered and balanced approach to allowing freedom for some risky behaviours but at the same time looking at ways to manage them in a supportive and safe environment.

> **Key points**
>
> - Empowering approaches should be facilitated as much as possible, allowing people to take greater control of their own lives.
> - Risk assessment should be about balancing harms and benefits. It is worth considering here whether it is the former or the latter which drive approaches in risk management.
> - Professional judgements need to address what exactly the nature of the problem is, where the problem is located and who is best placed to respond to the problem.
> - Communication is essential to the assessment process where knowledge of a person's previous social history and present interpretations can allow us to engage in their world and reality, rather then compel them into ours.

References

Audit Commission (2002) *Forget Me Not 2002. Developing Mental Health Services for Older People in England.* London: Audit Commission.

Beauchamp, T.L. (2000) The philosophical basis of psychiatric ethics, in S. Bloch, P. Chodoff and S. Green (eds) *Psychiatric Ethics*, 3rd edn. New York: Oxford University Press.

Beauchamp, T.L. and Childress, J.F. (2001) *Principles of Biomedical Ethics*, 5th edn. New York: Oxford University Press.

Bond, J., Corner, L., Lilley, A. and Ellwood, C. (2002) Medicalization of insight and caregivers' responses to risk in dementia, *Dementia*, 1: 313–28.

Bucks, R.S., Ashworth, D.L., Wilcock, G.K. and Siegfried, K. (1996) Assessment of activities of daily living in dementia: development of the Bristol Activities of Daily Living Scale, *Age and Ageing*, 25: 113–20.

Canter, R. (2001) Patients and medical power, *British Medical Journal*, 323 (7310), 414.

Clarke, C. (2000) Risk: constructing care and care environments in dementia, *Health, Risk and Society*, 2(1): 83–92.

Commission for Healthcare Audit and Inspection (2006) *Living Well into Later Life: A Review of Progress Against the National Service Framework for Older People.* London: Healthcare Commission.

DoH (Department of Health) (1991) *Care Management and Assessment: Practitioner's Guide.* London: DoH and Social Services Inspectorate.

DoH (Department of Health) (2000) *The NHS Plan.* London: NHS Executive, DoH.

DoH (Department of Health) (2009) *Living Well with Dementia: A New Dementia Strategy.* London: DoH.

Dowie, J. (1999) Communication for better decisions: not about risk, *Health, Risk and Society*, 1: 41–53.

Eckes, L.M. (1996) Active listening, *Gasteroenterology Nursing*, 6: 219–20.

Edwards, H. and Noller, P. (1998) Factors influencing caregiver – care receiver communication and its impact on the well-being of older care receivers, *Health Communication*, 10(4): 317–41.

Farsides, B. (2002) An ethical perspective – consent and patient autonomy, in J. Tingle and A. Cribb (eds) *Nursing Law and Ethics*, 2nd edn. Oxford: Blackwell Sciences.

Fulford, K.W.M. (1995) *Moral Theory and Medical Practice*, 2nd edn. Cambridge: Cambridge University Press.

Ganzini, L., Volicer, L., Nelson, W.A., Fox, E. and Dearse, A.R. (2004) Ten myths about decision-making capacity, *Journal of the American Medical Directors Association*, 5: 263–7.

Gerrish, K. (2001) The nature and effect of communication difficulties arising from interactions between district nurses and South Asian patients and their carers, *Journal of Advanced Nursing*, 33: 566–74.

Gibson, C.H. (1991) A concept analysis of empowerment, *Journal of Advanced Nursing*, 16(3): 354–61.

Goldsmith, M. (1996) *Hearing the Voices of People with Dementia: Opportunities and Obstacles*. London: Jessica Kinglsey.

Gordon. P. (1999) *Face to Face: Therapy as Ethics*. London: Constable.

Gunstone, S. (2003) Risk assessment and management of patients with self-neglect: a grey area for mental health workers, *Journal of Psychiatric and Mental Health*, 10(3): 287–96.

Harris, P. and Sterin, G. (1999) Insider's perspective: defining and preserving the self in dementia, *Journal of Mental Health and Aging*, 5: 241–56.

Health Service Ombudsman for England (2003) *HSC Annual Report 2002–3*. London: Health Service Ombudsman for England.

HPC (Health Professionals Council) (2002) *Working with Health Professionals to Protect the Public*, http://www.hpc-uk.org, accessed 12 December 2008.

Lamond, D., Crow, R. and Chase, J. (1996) Judgements and processes in care decisions in acute medical and surgical wards, *Journal of Evaluation in Clinical Practice*, 31(4): 214–16.

Lord Chancellor's Department (1999) *Making Decisions: The Government's Proposals for Making Decisions on Behalf of Mentally Incapacitated Adults*, CM4465. London: The Stationery Office.

Lubinski, R. (1991) *Dementia and Communication*. Philadelphia, PA: B.C. Decker.

Miller, L. (2002) Effective communication with older people, *Nursing Standard*, 17(9): 45–50.

NMC (Nursing and Midwifery Council) (2008) Code of *Professional Conduct: Standards for Conduct, Performance and Ethics*. London: NMC.

Palvianen, P., Hietala, M., Routasalo, P., Suominen, T. and Hupli, M. (2003) Do nurses exercise power in basic care situations? *Nursing Ethics*, 10(3): 269–80.

Parker, M. and Dickenson, D. (2001) *The Cambridge Medical Ethics Workbook*. Cambridge: Cambridge University Press.

Pearlin, L.I., Harrington, C., Montgomery, R.J.V. and Zarit, S.H. (2001) An overview of the social and behavioural consequences of Alzheimer's disease, *Aging and Mental Health*, 5(supplement 1): 3–6.

Pritchard, J. (1997) Vulnerable people taking risks: older people and residential care, in H. Kemshall and J. Pritchard (eds) *Good Practice in Risk and Risk Management 2: Protection, Rights and Responsibilities*. London: Jessica Kinglsey.

Reed, J. (1998) Care and protection of older people, in B. Heyman (ed.) *Risk, Health and Health Care: A Qualitative Approach*. London: Arnold.

Reisberg, B., Ferris, S., deLeon, M. and Crook, T. (1982) The global deterioration for assessment of primary degenerative dementia, *American Journal of Psychiatry*, 139: 1136–9.

Reisberg, B., Borenstein, J., Salob, S.P., Ferris, S.H., Franseen, E. and Georgotas, A. (1987) Behavioural symptoms in Alzheimer's disease: phenomenology and treatment, *Journal of Clinical Psychiatry*, 48(supplement 5): 9–15.

Royal Society (1992) *Risk: Analysis, Perception, Management. Report of a Royal Society Study Group*. London: The Royal Society.

Sabat, S. and Harré, R. (1992) The construction and deconstruction of self in Alzheimer's disease, *Ageing and Society*, 12: 443–61.

Thakerar, J., Giles, H. and Cheshire, J. (1982) Psychological and linguistic parameters of speech accommodation theory, in C. Fraser and K. Scherer (eds) *Advances in the Social Psychology of Language*. Cambridge: Cambridge University Press.

Wise, R. (2003) Language systems in normal and aphasic human subjects: functional imaging studies and inferences from animal studies, *British Medical Bulletin*, 65: 95–119.

Woods, B. and Pratt, R. (2005) Awareness in dementia: ethical and legal issues in relation to people with dementia, *Aging and Mental Health*, 9(5): 423–9.

9 Facilitating person-centred care: worksheets and activities

Objections: After reading this chapter you should be able to:

- Discuss how classroom discussions and activities can promote/maintain positive and realistic expectations towards the person with dementia and the care provided.
- Reflect upon how the use of experiential learning exercises can assist in individual and group awareness of issues relevant to dementia care.
- Explore the use of various experiential learning exercises within your practice area.

Introduction

This chapter explores some of the approaches which can be used to facilitate learning about dementia care. It is divided into two distinct parts, the first addressing some general themes with regards to the learning process and the second offering some specific exercises which can be used as part of a student learning or staff training programme.

The learning process

We all learn in different ways. Some of us gain more understanding from reading and individual reflection while others learn more effectively by actively taking part in group-based activities. Each person has their own set of life experiences, attitudes and understanding, and ways of working with the person with dementia. These incorporate both positive and negative views which might have been influenced through previous practice or by what has been picked up from peers or media sources. The challenge for educationalists is to explore some of the misconceptions about dementia and consider ways of working that can overcome the pessimism or stigma with which it is often associated. Such an approach fundamentally addresses ways in which students can contribute towards improving the quality of life of people with dementia.

This chapter offers a series of group-based experiential learning exercises that can be used within classroom teaching or as part of a staff training programme. The model of experiential learning (see Figure 9.1) developed by Kolb (1984) suggests that the process of learning consists of four phases:

1   *Concrete experience* (occurring when the person is involved in carrying out a task).
2   *Reflection* (a personal reflection on that experience).
3   *Abstract conceptualization* (identifying general rules and applying known theories leading to ideas about modifying the next occurrence of the experience).
4   *Active experimentation* (application of new skills or ideas into practice, leading to a new set of experiences which are in turn reflected on).

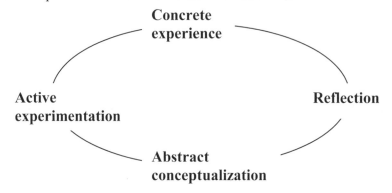

Figure 9.1   Experiential learning (Kolb 1984)

Through the teaching of dementia care to numerous healthcare students over many years we have developed a series of learning activities which facilitated personal reflection and promoted group discussion. The *ground rules* for the learning experience were negotiated with students and focused upon *acceptable* and *unacceptable* behaviours, examples of which can be found in Box 9.1.

Box 9.1 Ground rules

Acceptable

- Showing respect
- Maintaining confidentiality
- Listening to each other
- Being non-judgemental
- Offering constructive feedback
- Being punctual

Unacceptable

- Talking over each other
- Poor time-keeping
- Not listening
- Showing intolerance towards each other
- Being rude

As well as the experiential exercises detailed below we also offered healthcare students a series of day-long workshops that collectively explored 'ways of working' with individuals who had dementia and the variety of roles that professional carers could engage in. This incorporated an exploration of the culture of care that exists within clinical teams and the degree of optimism or pessimism that is subsequently promoted. While examining this, the subsequent impact that it had on the student's approach to care was reflected upon.

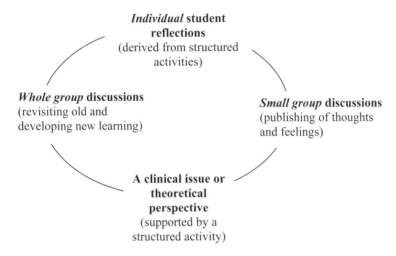

Figure 9.2 Practice reflections

One of the approaches we employed within the classroom environment (as outlined in Figure 9.2) was a *self–theory–self* format. The use of this learning cycle allows an event to be selected for reflection and a record of the experience to be kept. Using this record, the student's experience can be analysed in terms of what happened and why, what was expected to happen and what it means. Schön (1991) argued that professionals in their everyday practice face unique and complex situations that are unsolvable by adopting technical rational approaches alone, proposing an approach where professionals' learning is facilitated by reflection. This process was assisted through providing a range of structured activities and insight-building learning opportunities where students could reflect upon their own thoughts and feelings about working in dementia care and match these against the interpretations offered by peers. Boud and Walker (1998) state that reflection should enable learners to express doubts, uncertainty and awareness of contradictions. The 'publishing' of their interpretations within small groups encourages personal declarations and listening to reflections by peers. From this point of self-awareness, the inclusion of a contemporary healthcare concern asks the student to consider ways of integrating theoretical issues with practice. The importance of self-awareness is the space provided to analyse one's feelings honestly and to examine how the situation has affected the individual as well as how the individual has affected the situation (Schön 1991). This process encouraged students to acknowledge how their contributions and raised self-awareness could greatly benefit the individuals with dementia they engaged with.

With all the varied complexities of care, students were encouraged to keep a focus on the person within the condition of dementia. This occasionally caused frustration where students were placed with healthcare teams who seemed to predominantly deal with symptoms and behavioural manifestations as opposed to the person within the condition. The main approach here was to try and work around or within the obstacles and limitations presented and achieve the 'best fit' possible between idealized care and actual practice. This highlights the essence of this workbook which attempts to promote the best person-centred care possible despite the environmental, personal or professional constraints encountered.

The following section provides fuller details of the exercises outlined within each of the chapters. It details both the resources and structure for running these exercises and also offers some variations which could be considered as well.

Exercises

Chapter 2

Exercise 1: Watching *Iris*

Aim

This exercise is concerned with the impact of dementia on a married couple. Participants are able to witness how the writer Iris Murdoch (who had Alzheimer's disease) and her husband John Bayley lived within the shadow of dementia, and how her condition influenced their personal lives and relationship together.

Resources

- The film *Iris* (2001) starring Judy Dench and Jim Broadbent.
- Worksheet.

Worksheet

1   Before watching the film

What do I feel could be the felt/lived experience of people who have dementia?

2   While watching the film

What sense do we get of Iris and her felt experience?

What do we understand about her husband John's experience?

What do we learn of the impact the condition of dementia has upon their relationship?

3   After watching the film

To what degree have my values, beliefs and attitudes been influenced by watching this film?

What do we learn of the impact that the condition of dementia has upon a couple's relationship?

Activity

Participants are given a worksheet and asked to write responses to the first section considering their initial thoughts and feelings about what a person with dementia might be experiencing. During the viewing of Iris they are asked to consider the questions in section 2 and to note down their observations. After watching the film they are given an opportunity to sum up their thoughts about the ways that dementia can impact upon individuals and their relationships with partners. Space for discussion and a sharing of personal reflections with peers can follow, thereby maximizing learning.

Variations

Other films such as *The Notebook* (2004), *Away from Her* (2006) or *The Road to Galveston* (1996) could be used. These could be shown in their entirety or in selected clips in order to promote further discussion and reflection concerning the experience of dementia. Worksheet questions could be modified accordingly to address the particular issues reflected by each film.

Exercise 2: Understanding behaviour

Aim

This exercise encourages participants to become more aware of the inner thoughts and feelings about people with dementia. There are also opportunities to explore some of the underlying causes of 'challenging' behaviours observed in people with dementia.

Resources

- Book chapter 'The abnormal changes so far' in *My Journey into Alzheimer's Disease* (1989) by Robert Davis.
- Worksheet.

Worksheet

What sense do you make of the difficulties experienced by the narrator?

How might these affect his subsequent behaviour or response towards others?

Consider ways in which he could be best supported to cope with these difficulties.

Activity

Participants are given the chapter 'The abnormal changes so far' from Robert Davis's book *My Journey into Alzheimer's Disease* to read and asked to complete the accompanying worksheet. This chapter focuses specifically on some of the difficulties he was experiencing including paranoia, fear of making mistakes, poor concentration, agitation and wandering behaviour. Reading this chapter provides participants with an awareness of the inner thoughts and feelings that impact upon such behaviours, including those which might be regarded by others as challenging behaviours. Written responses from the worksheet inform the subsequent discussion.

Variations

Alternative books which feature first-person accounts of dementia could be used here. These include:

- *Living in the Labyrinth* (1993) by Diana Friel McGowin.
- *Show Me the Way to Go Home* (1996) by Larry Rose.
- *Out of Mind* (1988) by J. Bernlef.
- *Dancing with Dementia* (2005) by Christine Bryden.

Chapter 3

Exercise 1:   Internet guided study – 'the lived experience of carers'

Aim

This exercise uses a guided study to help promote insights into the actual felt and lived experience of dementia as encountered by carers. Participants are directed to the internet site created by the health charity group healthtalkonline. This site provides information about the carer's role from a first-person perspective.

Resources

- Internet access.
- Worksheet.

Worksheet

Go to www.healthtalkonline.org and look for 'dementia' under the A–Z list of conditions

1   Sample interviews from the following:

- Signs of dementia
- Getting the diagnosis
- Treatment of Alzheimer's disease
- Becoming a carer
- Friends and family
- Wandering
- End of life

2   Take a look at the extra themes covered in the 'Full list of topics' link. These include:

- Residential care
  Arranging residential care
  Becoming a resident
- Difficult decisions
  Wandering
  Driving
  Money
  Self care
  Respect
  Living with change
  Complicated emotions
  End of life

Activity

Participants are first asked to consider what they think the carer's experiences might be. They are then given the worksheet and access to the website. Carers' interviews can be accessed in different formats, read as transcripts, listened to as audio files or watched as videos. On completion participants are led into a discussion of their thoughts about carers' felt and lived experiences.

Variations

A similar exercise could be employed by looking through selected carers' accounts in the Alzheimer's Society's *Living with Dementia* online magazine. This can be located at www.alzheimers.org.uk/site/scripts/documents.php?categoryID=200241.

Exercise 2:   A day in the life

Aim

This exercise enables participants to become more mindful of the daily experience engaged in by carers of those with dementia. The approach here follows the familiar magazine structure of a 'day in the life' and involves looking at three distinct parts of a carer's typical day – morning, afternoon and evening (night-time details are not requested here).

Resources

- Access to family carers of individuals with dementia.
- Diary structure: morning, afternoon, evening.

Activity

Participants and carers are prepared accordingly for this exercise (including making the carer's 'daily activities' account available). Following this, carers enter the group accompanied by a facilitator and introductions are made. The sharing of experience is broken into the three designated parts with opportunities for questions and discussion following each section. The activity comprises an interactive dialogue of approximately 40 minutes, initially between facilitator and carer, but then with opportunities given for group participants to ask questions and get involved. Sensitivity is needed throughout this exercise to prevent it from becoming an intrusive or intimidating process. Carers are subsequently debriefed and supported accordingly with later opportunities offered for feedback and discussion among the participants.

Variations

This exercise could include a fourth section – that of night-time – although sensitivity is needed here to prevent it becoming intrusive. A carer's dialogue that explores the experience of receiving a dementia diagnosis could also be incorporated.

Chapter 4

Exercise 1: Circle of concerns

Aim

This exercise is designed to enable participants to begin to redefine practice problems as 'achievable challenges' while also being offered positive support from peers. There is an encouragement to reflect upon and listen to potential worries or perceived obstacles to working within dementia care services. Although various degrees of optimism, pessimism and enthusiasm might be expressed, the main approach taken is to consider constructive suggestions to tackling problems.

Resources

- A small piece of paper given to each participant including those who are facilitating the exercise.
- Chairs arranged where possible into a circular pattern (to close the group) although if not possible then ensure that all members are able to see each other.

Activity

Each participant is asked to briefly write down a 'concern' they have about caring for a person with dementia. These 'concerns' are written anonymously, folded and placed in a pile which is then mixed up. Participants then randomly select a piece of paper and it doesn't matter if the original writer collects their own 'concern'. Each person in turn reads their statement so that the group have a chance hear what the 'concern' is. A structured approach is recommended, for example, following the first reading the person on the left continues. Once all the 'concerns' have been read the process is repeated but this time fellow participants are encouraged to give constructive and positive responses. This activity allows both individual and group reflection upon participants' 'concerns' about working in dementia care services.

Variations

The 'circle of concerns' activity can revisit the participants' initial issues at a later time during their clinical experience in order to reflect upon the following themes.

- The extent to which attitudes have changed.
- Whether original 'concerns' were still an issue.
- The ways in which participants tackled 'concerns' and made a difference to individuals with dementia and their carers.

Exercise 2: Age and ageism

Aim

This exercise intends to reflect upon participants' views about ageing. It provides opportunities to discuss how attitudes (either positive or negative) can be formed towards older people.

Resources

- Worksheet.

Worksheet

My thoughts and feelings about the age I am …

What I think about people who are 30 years older than me …

What age do you consider a person becomes 'old' and why?

Activity

Each participant is given a worksheet to complete. This is done individually with opportunities provided to share thoughts within small groups. Groups are established according to decade of birth, i.e. 1960s, 1970s, 1980s and 1990s. Discussions take place within decade groups first and are then shared with the wider group to compare generational differences. This offers space for participants to reflect upon differing thoughts and levels of comfort with regard to the concept of ageing.

Variations

Additional themes or questions could be included within the worksheet such as 'Do you think that younger generations would be able to sufficiently meet your needs when you are considered to be "old"?' and 'Realistically, how could you address concerns about ageist attitudes in the workplace?'

Chapter 5

Exercise 1: Marks of well-being

Aim

This exercise aims to look more critically at the factors highlighted by Kitwood and Bredin (1992) as being vital in helping to maintain a person's feeling of well-being.

Resources

- 12 strips of paper, each containing one of the identified 'Marks of Well-being'.
- Worksheet.

Worksheet

Marks of Well-being (Kitwood and Bredin 1992)

- Being able to assert one's own wills or desires
- Being able to express a range of emotions, of both happiness and distress
- Initiating contact with others
- Being affectionate
- Being sensitive to the needs and feelings of others
- Having self-respect
- Accepting other confused people
- Enjoying humour
- Self-expression, being creative
- Showing pleasure
- Being able to relax
- Helpfulness

Activity

Participants (in groups) are given the 'Marks of Well-being' items and asked to place them into three separate categories:

- Absolutely essential
- Very important
- Less important

Each group is given the task of providing a rationale for the placing of an item within a particular category which is then fed back to the wider group. This exercise can generate a fair degree of debate and conflicting opinions as to where certain items should be placed. Groups should be supported in their endeavours and reminded that there is not one ideal solution.

Variations

A similar process to that outlined above can be carried out with the 'Marks of Ill-being':

- Depressed or despairing
- Intensely angry or aggressive
- Shows anxiety or fear
- Agitated or restless
- Withdrawn or listless
- Has physical discomfort or pain
- Unresolved grieving over losses
- Bodily tension
- Easily 'walked over' by other people
- An outsider

Exercise 2:   Dimensions and the social environment

Aim

This exercise encourages participants to think about related issues when designing their own dementia care environment.

Resources

- Copies of Moos and Lemke's (1985) *Dimensions of Social Environment.*
- Worksheet.

Dimensions of social environment (Moos and Lemke 1985)

1   Relationships

- Integration – degree to which residents are integrated into the life of the home.
- Privacy – degree to which residents are able to separate from the community.

2   Personal growth

- Stimulation – degree to which residents are kept active and participating.
- Freedom – degree to which residents are free to use the facilities of the home or leave the home.
- Continuity – degree to which staff in the home have information on the resident's life history and links that are maintained with the past.

3   System maintenance and change

- Planned care – degree to which care plans and policies are thought through and discussed.
- Regimentation – degree to which care tasks take place at the convenience of staff rather than the individual needs/desires of residents.
- Control – degree to which residents have control over their lives.

Worksheet

You are designing a new residential facility for 20 women (over 65) with dementia

1 Show how you will accommodate the various aspects relating to:

- Relationships
- Personal growth
- System maintenance and change

2 In particular, how will you manage the competing needs of privacy and integration?

3 Which of the above aspects is the hardest to facilitate and why?

4 Show your design of the building (including layout, garden space, etc.).

5 How will carers' needs be accommodated?

Activity

This exercise encourages participants to explore ideas and intentions in designing an environment capable of meeting the needs of residents with dementia. Moos and Lemke's framework is used as a structure to consider related themes. Participants are placed in small groups and asked to address questions on the worksheet. Plans and thoughts are then related back to the wider group for discussion.

Variations

The same exercise can be used but this time with different groups of service users, for example males under 65, or a mixed-sex residency. Following this exercise, specific 'issues' can be given to participants to discuss, such as ways to accommodate a person's sexual needs, risky behaviours or their need to smoke or drink.

Chapter 6

Exercise 1:   Malignant social psychology (MSP)

Aim

This exercise helps participants to appreciate and recognize some of the pressures and difficulties that might lead to the delivery of poor care practices.

Resources

- Copies of Kitwood's (1997) 'malignant social psychology' factors (see Appendix 2 for further details).

Malignant social psychology (Kitwood 1997)

1   Treachery
2   Disempowerment
3   Infantilization
4   Intimidation
5   Labelling
6   Stigmatization
7   Outpacing
8   Invalidation
9   Banishment
10 Objectification
11 Ignoring
12 Imposition
13 Withholding
14 Accusation
15 Disruption
16 Mockery
17 Disparagement

Activity

This exercise engages participants to consider potential negative approaches that might be encountered in practice. The importance of this activity is to be aware of the pressures and difficulties experienced which might influence these approaches being used, even by otherwise caring and attentive staff. The following questions are addressed within small groups.

- What do you think causes approaches such as these to develop?
- Which of the 17 aspects is the most harmful and why?
- What might cause me to be drawn into any of these ways of responding?
- What can we do to limit and restrict their occurrence?

After receiving group feedback it should be acknowledged that while we might distance ourselves from such behaviours with the assumption that these are 'uncaring' practices, we need to recognize that we too can get drawn into using some of these responses without even noticing it.

Variations

Using the 'malignant social psychology' as a resource, develop a corresponding list of 'positive social psychology' factors and consider how these might be best maintained in practice.

Exercise 2:   Planning a reminiscence activity

Aim

This exercise is geared towards helping participants plan appropriate reminiscence work with individuals with dementia.

Resources

- Poster paper and pens.
- Worksheet.

Worksheet

Core focus

Finding positive memories – especially positive or productive for individuals where large areas of the past are dominated by painful experiences. This approach might for some entail an exclusive focus upon positive and pleasurable issues.

You will be placed in one of two groups relating to where you are currently working (see below).

- Community
- Inpatient

We are now taking you 50 years into the future and would like you to consider your fellow classmates as the potential clients for your reminiscence activity.

1   Plan a reminiscence activity which can be used either with a group in a healthcare setting or with individuals in their own homes. This activity is geared towards interaction, memory-sharing and individual recollection/identity strengthening

2   Describe the activity in detail including specific resources or examples you plan to use.

Activity

Healthcare students are placed into one of the following groups that relate to where they are currently working:

- Community (living at home or attending day care services)
- Inpatient (resident in a health service facility)

The groups having been established their remit is to plan 50 years into the future in order to consider the types of activity that would be appropriate if their colleagues were to become members in a reminiscence group. The preparation for this exercise could commence with a discussion about a number of current-day examples which despite being 'popular' (i.e. *Big Brother*) are not universally enjoyed or engaged in by all. The task for each of the groups is then to carefully select reminiscence materials which are likely to be favourably received in the future and to create positive feelings among the participants.

Variations

Look at *common* reminiscence approaches which are used in practice and discuss the criteria (or lack of) used in their selection and their appropriateness to those they are offered to.

Chapter 7

Exercise 1: Three circles

Aim

This exercise examines our engagement with people with dementia and the extent to which this is influenced by the degree of cognitive deterioration present. It looks essentially at our engagement with two separate components – P (the person) and D (the condition of dementia).

Resources

- Worksheet.

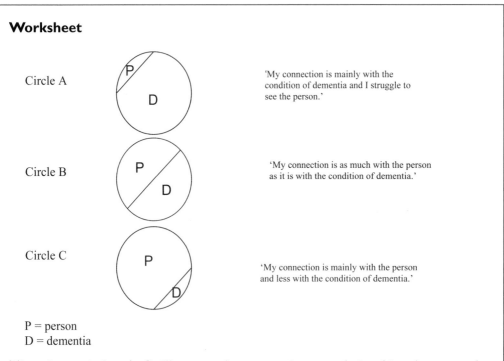

Worksheet

Circle A

'My connection is mainly with the condition of dementia and I struggle to see the person.'

Circle B

'My connection is as much with the person as it is with the condition of dementia.'

Circle C

'My connection is mainly with the person and less with the condition of dementia.'

P = person
D = dementia

The above circles A–C illustrate the proportionate relationships between the person being related to and the condition of dementia.

Chose an individual you are currently working with and consider which of the above relationships (A, B or C) best fits your approach.

Write down the rationale for your choice.

Activity

Participants are first encouraged to reflect upon a person they are currently working with or have had recent involvement with. The exercise worksheet is then given out and they are asked to consider which of the three circles A, B or C best fits the type of connection that is made. A rationale for their choice of circles should be stated. Opportunities for discussion and feedback should follow with particular attention given to occasions where the other types of engagement (not chosen here) can be experienced.

Variations

Identify all the approaches that help to affirm a person's personal identity. Participants are then asked to consider the value of this to the person with dementia and carers.

Exercise 2:   The language of dementia

Aim

This exercise aims to help participants become more aware about communication approaches that can be used when the verbal mode becomes impaired.

Resources

- Description cards ('What I want/don't want to wear'; 'What I want/don't want to eat for breakfast'; 'What I want/don't want to do today').
- Foreign language speakers.

Activity

Participants are divided into three groups of a) *persons with dementia*; b) *healthcare staff*: and c) *clinical supervisors*. The *persons with dementia* are selected from individuals who have a passing knowledge in any language other than English. Proper fluency is not required and participants are free to submit other words where certain translations are not known. *Persons with dementia* have time to prepare their responses – these should not be shown to *healthcare staff*. The requests are then made in another language directly to *healthcare staff* who have to try and ascertain what is being asked. Opportunities to 'freeze' the activity and consult with *clinical supervisors* are provided.

Variation

This exercise can be modified with activities being substituted by emotions. The *person with dementia* therefore talks about how they are feeling to *healthcare staff*.

Chapter 8

Exercise 1: Debating empowerment

Aim

This exercise explores participants' understanding of the term 'empowerment' and its potential benefits for the person with dementia. It also considers factors which might disempower a person and prevent them from being more autonomous. A debate is set up to consider the conflicting 'stances' or views encountered within practice.

Resources

- Poster paper.
- Debating positions A and B.
- Feedback sheets.

Activity

Three groups are formed who work out of earshot to discuss:

- Position A: why empowerment is important for the person with dementia
- Position B: why it is less risky and easier to do things for the person with dementia

Participants are allowed approximately 15 minutes to formulate their arguments which are written down as bullet points. They also construct a brief statement which forms their concluding remarks. The third group adopt an observer's role and offer feedback on the debating process. An example of their feedback sheet with points for observation is included below.

Empowerment feedback

empowerment	*disempowerment*
group	*group*
convincing arguments	
realistic rationales	
objective concluding remark	

Below is a suggested seating layout for the debate.

At any one time only 'active debaters' can become involved in the discussion and respective colleagues can take their place by tapping them on the shoulder. Allow approximately ten minutes for this part of the activity. The concluding part of the activity commences with the 'observers' offering comments from their feedback sheets on the contributions from both groups. Their feedback should stimulate discussions around the debate and the concluding thoughts of each group about the two different positions.

Variations

The three small groups are asked to look at the notion of empowerment as it relates to:

- Family carers
- Healthcare professionals
- Mental health advocacy groups

A debate can then be set up between these groups regarding their thoughts about the empowering process with those experiencing dementia.

Exercise 2: What makes risky behaviours?

Aim

This exercise considers how participants determine what behaviours could be deemed 'risky'. It commences with sharing aspects of their own lifestyles and a reminder about confidentiality needs to be included prior to disclosure. Discussions on the potential difficulties in agreeing a rating scale and how discrepancies in determining the degree of risk can be established.

Resources

- Paper/pens.
- Behaviour rating sheet.

Behaviour rating sheet		
0–3	4–7	8–10
behaviours		
•		
•		
•		
•		
•		

Activity

Participants are asked to identify any 'risky' behaviours they might have engaged in over the previous month. They are then allocated to work in pairs to discuss their behaviours. Following this a group presentation sheet is produced which informs the discussions on ways of assessing the degree of risky behaviours. Themes underpinning group discussions can include the following.

- What 'risk' is defined as and the extent to which it influences a person's ability to take risks.
- How consensus is arrived at in interpreting risky behaviours.
- The comparison between initial ratings of behaviour and group decisions.
- Issues of objectivity and subjectivity.

Variations

Ask participants to comment upon their observations/contributions in assessing a person's risk level. Consider how the individual's risk behaviours are viewed and decisions arrived at by health professionals within the clinical setting. With regards to practice experience, identify what the consequences of risk management are to the person with dementia.

References

Bernlef, J. (1988) *Out of Mind*. London: Faber & Faber.

Boud, D. and Walker, D. (1998) Promoting reflection in professional courses: the challenge of context, *Studies in Higher Education*, 23(2): 191–206.

Bryden, C. (2005) *Dancing with Dementia*. London: Jessica Kingsley.

Davis, R. (1989) *My Journey into Alzheimer's Disease*. Buckinghamshire: Tyndale House.

Friel-McGowin, D. (1993) *Living in the Labyrinth: A Personal Journey through the Maze of Alzheimer's Disease*. New York: Delacorte Press.

Kitwood, T. (1997) *Dementia Reconsidered*. Buckingham: Open University Press.

Kitwood, T. and Bredin, K. (1992) *Person-Person: A Guide to the Care of those with Failing Mental Powers*. Loughton: Gale Centre.

Kolb, D. (1984) *Experiential Learning Experience as the Source of Learning and Development*. Englewood Cliffs, NJ: Prentice-Hall.

Moos, R. and Lemke, S. (1985) Specialised living environments for older people, in J. Birren and K. Schaie (eds) *Handbook of the Psychology of Aging*. New York: Reinhold.

Rose, L. (1996) *Show Me the Way to Go Home*. Forest Knolls, CA: Elder Books.

Schön, D. (1991) *The Reflective Practitioner*, 2nd edn. San Francisco, CA: Jossey Bass.

Appendix 1: Dementia websites

This section includes a selection of current websites which are concerned with the topic of dementia. A website address and brief summary of each is provided – these have been placed within the following categories:

- Services and organizations
- Documents and reports.

Services and organizations

Alzheimer's Association

www.alz.org/AboutAD/Stages.asp

This site provides information by the leading voluntary health organization in the USA for Alzheimer's care.

Alzheimer's Disease International

www.alz.co.uk/carers/yourself.html

Alzheimer's Disease International (ADI) is the umbrella organization of Alzheimer associations around the world. Its aim is to help establish and strengthen Alzheimer associations globally and to raise awareness about Alzheimer's disease and all other causes of dementia.

Alzheimer's Research Trust

www.alzheimers-research.org.uk/

The Alzheimers Research Trust is the leading UK research charity for dementia and funds world-class research to find ways to cure, prevent or treat Alzheimer's disease and related dementias.

Alzheimer's Scotland

www.alzscot.org/

This is the website of Scotland's leading voluntary organization helping people with dementia and their carers and families.

Alzheimer's Society

www.alzheimers.org.uk/site/index.php

The Alzheimer's Society is the leading UK care and research charity for people with dementia, their families and carers.

atdementia

www.atdementia.org.uk/

atdementia provides user-friendly information on assistive technology for people with dementia including what is available and how it can be obtained.

Bradford Dementia Group

www.brad.ac.uk/acad/health/dementia/

This group aims to improve the quality of life and care for people with dementia and their families, through excellence in research, education and training.

Dementia Advocacy Support Network International

www.dasninternational.org

This is a worldwide support network established in 2000 to promote respect and dignity, encourage support mechanisms and advocate on behalf of people with dementia.

Dementia Café

www.dementiacafe.com/news.php

The Dementia Café is a place for people with dementia, their carers and professionals to talk, share information, get advice and generally offer support to each other.

Mental Health Foundation

www.mentalhealth.org.uk/information/mental-health-a-z/dementia/

The Mental Health Foundation provides useful information and links to related research and publications concerning dementia and its care.

Telecare

www.telecare.org.uk/information/45763/home/

This is the website for the Telecare Services Association which is designed to help service users, their carers and families to learn more about Telecare services and products.

Documents and reports

A New Ambition for Old Age

www.dh.gov.uk/en/Publicationsandstatistics/Publications/
PublicationsPolicyAndGuidance/DH_4133941

The priorities for the second phase of the government's ten-year National Service Framework (NSF) for Older People are set out here under three themes: dignity in care, joined-up care and healthy ageing.

Dementia: Out of the Shadows

www.alzheimers.org.uk/downloads/Out_of_the_Shadows.pdf

People with dementia speak out about the impact stigma and diagnosis have on their lives in this Alzheimer's Society report.

Dementia: Supporting People with Dementia and their Carers in Health and Social Care

http://guidance.nice.org.uk/download.aspx?o=CG42PublicInfoWord

This booklet from NICE (the National Institute for Health and Clinical Excellence) is written for people with dementia and their carers about the support and treatment of people with dementia.

Dignity in Care

www.dh.gov.uk/en/Policyandguidance/Healthandsocialcaretopics/Socialcare/
Dignityincare/index.htm

The Dignity in Care campaign aims to put dignity at the heart of care and create a care system where there is zero tolerance of abuse and disrespect of older people.

Everybody's Business: Integrated Mental Health Services for Older Adults: A Service Development Guide

http://olderpeoplesmentalhealth.csip.org.uk/everybodys-business.html

Everybody's Business aims at improving health and social care practice with particular emphasis upon older people's mental health.

Inquiry into Mental Health and Well-being in Later Life

www.mhilli.org/

This inquiry was set up to raise awareness of mental health and well-being in later life, involving and empowering older people as well as creating better understanding, influencing policy and planning, and improving services.

Living Well in Later Life

www.audit-commission.gov.uk/Products/NATIONAL-REPORT/4C4C40BE-6383–
40E0–8B26–48D7FAF39A56/HCC_older%20PeopleREP.pdf

This document reviews the progress made concerning The National Service Framework for Older People.

Living Well with Dementia: A New Dementia Strategy

www.dh.gov.uk/en/Publicationsandstatistics/Publications/
PublicationsPolicyAndGuidance/DH_094058

This strategy provides a framework within which local services can deliver quality improvements to dementia services and address health inequalities relating to dementia.

Living with Dementia magazine

www.alzheimers.org.uk/site/scripts/documents.php?categoryID=200241

This online magazine is the the monthly national newsletter of the Alzheimer's Society.

Mental Capacity Act 2005

www.dca.gov.uk/menincap/bill-summary.htm

This Act provides a statutory framework to empower and protect vulnerable people who may not be able to make their own decisions. It makes it clear who can take decisions, in which situations, and how they should go about it. It also enables people to plan ahead for a time when they may lose capacity.

National Service Framework for Older People

www.dh.gov.uk/en/Publicationsandstatistics/Publications/
PublicationsPolicyAndGuidance/DH_4003066

The National Service Framework for Older People was established to look at the problems older people face in receiving care in order to deliver higher quality services.

NICE

www.nice.org.uk

This site contains information from the independent organization responsible for providing national guidance for healthcare. It includes recommendations concerning prescribing medication for those with dementia.

Securing Better Mental Health for Older Adults

www.dh.gov.uk/en/Publicationsandstatistics/Publications/
PublicationsPolicyAndGuidance/DH_4114989

This document provides a vision for how all mainstream health and social care services, with the support of specialist services, should work together to secure better mental health for older adults.

Supporting People with Long Term Conditions

www.dh.gov.uk/en/Publicationsandstatistics/Publications/
PublicationsPolicyAndGuidance/DH_4100252

This model looks at ways to help local health communities in developing a more integrated and systematic approach to care for people with long-term conditions.

Transforming the Quality of Dementia Care

www.dh.gov.uk/en/Consultations/Liveconsultations/DH_085570

The Department of Health's proposed national strategy for dementia services aims at improving awareness of dementia, ensuring that the condition is diagnosed as early as possible and delivering a high quality of care and support for those with dementia and their carers.

Appendix 2:
Malignant social psychology

1 **Treachery** – using forms of deception in order to distract or manipulate a person, or force them into compliance.

2 **Disempowerment** – not allowing a person to use the abilities that they do have; failing to help them complete actions they have initiated.

3 **Infantilization** – treating a person patronizingly as an insensitive parent might a very young child.

4 **Intimidation** – inducing fear in a person, through the use of threats or physical power.

5 **Labelling** – using a category such as dementia as the main basis for interacting with a person and for explaining their behaviour.

6 **Stigmatization** – treating a person as if they were a diseased object, an alien or outcast.

7 **Outpacing** – proving information and presenting choices at a rate too fast for a person to understand; putting them under pressure to do things more rapidly than they can bear.

8 **Invalidation** – failing to acknowledge the subjective reality of a person's experience and especially what they are feeling.

9 **Banishment** – sending a person away, or excluding them, physically or psychologically.

10 **Objectification** – treating a person as if they were a lump of dead matter, to be pushed, lifted, filled, pumped or drained without proper reference to the fact that they are sentient beings.

11 **Ignoring** – carrying on conversations or actions in the presence of a person as if they were not there.

12 **Imposition** – forcing a person to do something; denying choice on their part.

13 **Withholding** – refusing to give asked for-attention, or to meet an evident need.

14 **Accusation** – blaming a person for actions or failures of action that arise from their lack of ability, or their misunderstanding of the situation.

15 **Disruption** – intruding suddenly or disturbingly upon a person's action or reflection; crudely breaking their frame of reference.

16 **Mockery** – making fun of a person's actions or remarks; teasing, humiliating, making jokes at their expense.

17 **Disparagement** – telling a person they are incompetent, useless, worthless.

Source: Kitwood, T. (1997) *Dementia Reconsidered*. Buckingham: Open University Press.

Index

TOM KITWOOD ON DEMENTIA

A Reader and Critical Commentary

Clive Baldwin and Andrea Capstick

- How does Kitwood's work contribute to our understanding of 'the dementing process' and the essentials of quality care?
- How was Kitwood's thinking about dementia influenced by the wider context of his work in theology, psychology and biochemistry?
- What is the relevance today of key themes and issues in Kitwood's work?

Tom Kitwood was one of the most influential writers on dementia of the last 20 years. Key concepts and approaches from his work on person-centred care and well-being in dementia have gained international recognition and shaped much current thinking about practice development. The complexities of Kitwood's work and the development of his thinking over time have, however, received less attention. This Reader brings together twenty original publications by Kitwood which span the entire period of his writing on dementia, and the different audiences for whom he wrote.

Almost ten years after Kitwood's death, it is now timely to review his contribution to the field of dementia studies in the light of more recent developments and from a critical and interdisciplinary perspective. The introduction to this Reader summarises and problematises some of the key characteristics of Kitwood's writing. Each of the four themed sections begins with a commentary offering a balanced consideration of the strengths of Kitwood's work, but also of its limitations and oversights. The Reader also includes a biography and annotated bibliography.

Tom Kitwood on Dementia: A Reader and Critical Commentary is key reading for students of social work or mental health nursing, with an interest in dementia care. Professionals working with people with dementia will also find it invaluable.

Additional Contributors: Habib Chaudhury, Deborah O'Connor, Alison Phinney, Barbara Purves, Ruth Bartlett.

Contents: *Acknowledgements – About the Editors – Introduction – Section 1: Critique of the standard paradigm – Section 2: Ill-being, well-being and psychological need – Section 3: Personhood – Section 4: Organisational culture and its transformation – Bibliography – References.*

2007   384pp
978-0-335-22271-1 (Paperback)   978-0-335-22272-8 (Hardback)

Mental Health and Well Being in Later Life

Mima Cattan

"This book's main contribution … is to say to us all there is no single solution, no magic bullet, no instant cure, for the discomforts and illnesses of older age, and that not all ageing is comfortable. But it also tells us that it is in our control to do something about much of this, that older people's mental well-being could be vastly improved, and that public policy, and private attitudes, need to change. I hope that it is as influential as it deserves to be."

Taken from the foreword by Baroness Julia Neuberger, Former Chief Executive of the King's Fund and author of 'Not Dead Yet'

Mental health issues amongst older adults are becoming ever more prevalent. This fascinating book looks broadly at the mental health and well being issues that affect adults in later life. Taking a holistic approach to mental health and mental health promotion, the book explores the debates around what is meant by mental health and mental illness and the wider social determinants of mental health.

All chapters have a common thread running through them – each of which was identified as being a key theme for mental health and well-being by adults in later life. Among them are issues relating to:

- Gender
- Ethnicity
- Societal diversity
- Poverty
- Class
- Cultural differences

A range of examples from the UK and other countries, along with insights gained from older people's own perspectives, are used to emphasise the evidence base for effective interventions to promote mental health. Case studies, vignettes and quotes demonstrate how social theory and principles of health promotion can be effectively applied to improve practice.

Mental Health and Well Being in Later Life is key reading for those working or intending to work in public health, health promotion and health and social care professions, especially those who work with older people.

Contents: Introduction – What is mental health and mental well-being – Theoretical perspectives of ageing and health promotion – The application of policy and practice in the promotion of mental health and well-being in later life – Work, retirement and money – Relationships – Keeping active [physically and mentally] – Maintaining capability – Retaining independence and control

2009   184pp
ISBN-13: 978-0-335-22892-8   (ISBN-10: 0335-2-2892-5) Paperback
ISBN-13: 978-0-335-22891-1   (ISBN-10: 0335-2-2891-7) Hardback

EXCELLENCE IN DEMENTIA CARE

Research into Practice

Murna Downs and Barbara Bowers (eds)

'Dementia care has come of age with this book. It is an impeccably crafted collection of papers from eminent experts on both sides of the Atlantic. The book demonstrates confidence, based on both research evidence and well-grounded good practice, and a solid set of shared values both explicit and implicit. The contributors are refreshingly candid about debates and controversies. This book is authoritative and readable which makes it useful to a wide audience. It will provide knowledge, encouragement and motivation to a hard pressed workforce.'

Mary Marshall OBE, Emeritus Professor, University of Stirling, Scotland

This landmark textbook draws on the extensive knowledge of researchers, practitioners, and professionals in the care of people with Alzheimer's disease and other dementias. It is informed both by a profound respect for people with dementia and a commitment to including them in decisions about their care and lives. While focusing on care for people with dementia, this core text also addresses the most pressing concerns of families by promoting practices and services that recognise the full humanity of their relative with dementia. In addressing the many complex issues related to offering support to people with dementia and those who care for them, this timely textbook is unique in emphasising strategies for creating sustainable change in practice. The book includes examples from a range of countries, drawn from research, practice wisdom and, most importantly, from the experience of people with dementia and their families.

This key text offers valuable insights about how to:

- Provide competent and compassionate care for people with Alzheimer's Disease and other dementias
- Build systems to provide effective care
- Encourage collaboration among multi disciplinary professionals and users and carers
- Support those caring for people with dementia
- Ensure those with dementia maintain dignity, well-being and meaningful participation in life

Excellence in Dementia Care is a vital resource for those working with people with dementia. It provides an accessible yet sophisticated overview of the knowledge, skills and attitudes required to achieve excellence. It is an essential handbook for those responsible for training, education and skills development in dementia care.

Contents: *Contributors – Foreword – Preface – Acknowledgements – Introduction – Part 1: Principles and perspectives – Prevalence and projections of dementia – Toward understanding subjective experiences of dementia – Ethnicity and the experience of dementia – A bio-psycho-social approach to dementia – Flexibility and change: the fundamentals for families coping with dementia – Towards a person-centred ethic in dementia care: doing right or being good? – Being minded in dementia: persons and human beings – Part 2: Knowledge and skills for supporting people with dementia – Assessment and dementia – Supporting cognitive abilities – Working with life history – The language of behaviour – Communication and relationships: an inclusive social world – Supporting health and physical well-being – Understanding and alleviating emotional distress – Part 3: Journeys through dementia care – Diagnosis and early support – Living at home – Care of people with dementia in the general hospital – The role of specialist housing in supporting people with dementia – Care homes – End of life care – Grief and bereavement – Part 4: Embedding excellence in dementia care – Involving people with dementia in service development and evaluation – A trained and supported workforce – Attending to relationships in dementia care – Leadership in dementia care – Quality: the perspective of the person with dementia – Reframing dementia: the policy implications of changing concepts – The history and impact of dementia care policy – Index.*

2008   640pp

978-0-335-22375-6 (Paperback) 978-0-335-22374-9 (Hardback)